100 Questions & About Deep Vein Thrombosis and Pulmonary Embolism

Andra H. James, MD

Director, Women's Hemostasis and Thrombosis Clinic
Assistant Professor of Obstetrics and Gynecology
Duke University Medical Center, Durham, NC

Thomas L. Ortel, MD, PhD

Associate Professor of Medicine & Pathology
Director, Duke Hemostasis & Thrombosis Center
Duke University Health System, Durham, NC

Victor F. Tapson, MD

Professor of Medicine
Division of Pulmonary and Critical Care
Director, Center for Pulmonary Vascular Disease
Duke University Medical Center, Durham, NC

JONES AND BARTLETT PUBLISHERS
Sudbury, Massachusetts
BOSTON   TORONTO   LONDON   SINGAPORE

World Headquarters
Jones and Bartlett Publishers
40 Tall Pine Drive
Sudbury, MA 01776
978-443-5000
info@jbpub.com
www.jbpub.com

Jones and Bartlett Publishers
Canada
6339 Ormindale Way
Mississauga, Ontario L5V 1J2
CANADA

Jones and Bartlett Publishers
International
Barb House, Barb Mews
London W6 7PA
UK

Jones and Bartlett's books and products are available through most bookstores and online booksellers. To contact Jones and Bartlett Publishers directly, call 800-832-0034, fax 978-443-8000, or visit our website, www.jbpub.com.

Substantial discounts on bulk quantities of Jones and Bartlett's publications are available to corporations, professional associations, and other qualified organizations. For details and specific discount information, contact the special sales department at Jones and Bartlett via the above contact information or send an email to specialsales@jbpub.com.

The authors, editor, and publisher have made every effort to provide accurate information. However, they are not responsible for errors, omissions, or for any outcomes related to the use of the contents of this book and take no responsibility for the use of the products and procedures described. Treatments and side effects described in this book may not be applicable to all people; likewise, some people may require a dose or experience a side effect that is not described herein. Drugs and medical devices are discussed that may have limited availability controlled by the Food and Drug Administration (FDA) for use only in a research study or clinical trial. Research, clinical practice, and government regulations often change the accepted standard in this field. When consideration is being given to use of any drug in the clinical setting, the health care provider or reader is responsible for determining FDA status of the drug, reading the package insert, and reviewing prescribing information for the most up-to-date recommendations on dose, precautions, and contraindications, and determining the appropriate usage for the product. This is especially important in the case of drugs that are new or seldom used.

Production Credits
Executive Publisher: Chris Davis
Production Director: Amy Rose
Associate Production Editor: Rachel Rossi
Associate Editor: Kathy Richardson
Senior Marketing Manager: Katrina Gosek
Associate Marketing Manager: Rebecca Wasley

Manufacturing Buyer: Amy Bacus
Composition: Appingo
Cover Design: Jon Ayotte
Printing and Binding: Malloy, Inc.
Cover Printing: Malloy, Inc.

Library of Congress Cataloging-in-Publication Data
James, Andra H.
  100 questions & answers about deep vein thrombosis and pulmonary embolism / Andra H. James, Victor F. Tapson, Thomas L. Ortel.
    p. cm.
  Includes index.
  ISBN-13: 978-0-7637-4105-1 (alk. paper)
  ISBN-10: 0-7637-4105-1 (alk. paper)
  1. Thrombophlebitis. 2. Pulmonary embolism. I. Tapson, Victor F. II. Ortel, Thomas L. (Thomas Lee), 1957- III. Title. IV. Title: One hundred questions and answers about deep vein thrombosis and pulmonary embolism.
  RC696.J36 2008
  616.1'42--dc22
                    2007003325
6048

Printed in the United States of America
11 10 09 08 07   10 9 8 7 6 5 4 3 2 1

CONTENTS

According to the *American Heart Association 2007 Heart Disease and Stroke Statistics*, venous thromboembolism (VTE), including deep vein thrombosis (DVT), and pulmonary embolism (PE), occurs in nearly 100 per 100,000 persons in the United States each year. This, in turn, translates to greater than 200,000 new cases of VTE yearly, with increased rates among the elderly, obese individuals, persons sustaining a stroke, and in the setting of cancer and its treatment. Nationwide directives orchestrated by the *National Quality Forum* and *Joint Commission on Accreditation of Health Care Organizations* have reduced the number of VTEs occurring among hospitalized patients through education, risk assessment, and preventive measures. Nevertheless, an opportunity for improvement remains evident.

A statistics-oriented view of VTE, while important for assessing national health problems, evaluating relevant trends, and establishing a platform for both natural history-altering research and advocacy, does not capture fully the deeply personal side of the problem; it fails to project the real-life stories of Dena, Jennifer, Marvin, David, Michael, and Lori; and it falls well short of truly understanding VTE from the inside. Indeed, VTE is an affliction of people like you and me; people with jobs, people with friends and family, and people with dreams. *100 Questions & Answers about Deep Vein Thrombosis and Pulmonary Embolism* is a book about people written by three knowledgeable, experienced, compassionate, and caring physicians: Drs. James, Tapson, and Ortel, who commit themselves daily to people living with VTE. Their message is designed to inform; their words are crafted to reassure, enlighten, and empower, and their overriding, collective, and unconditional purpose is to heal.

Richard C. Becker, MD
Professor of Medicine
Divisions of Hematology and Cardiovascular Medicine
Duke University School of Medicine

We were invited to write this book, *100 Questions & Answers about Deep Vein Thrombosis and Pulmonary Embolism,* by Chris Davis, Executive Publisher at Jones and Bartlett and we seized the opportunity. We often said that we should create a series of brochures, or other written materials, to answer the questions we most commonly receive from patients and their family members. Now we have assembled these questions and answers in one book. We have tried to answer the types of questions that newly diagnosed patients ask, such as, "Why did I have this blood clot?" and "How can I get rid of it?", as well as the questions that patients ask later such as "What does this mean for my family members?", "How do I maintain my lifestyle?", and "How can I avoid having another blood clot?" We have tried to answer the questions using conversational English as opposed to medical terms, and where we have used medical terms, we have tried to define and explain them. This book has been written so each question and answer can be read individually, so that the book can be used as a reference, or so that the book can be read in its entirety, if desired. While the recommendations in the book should not be substituted for the guidance of one's physician or healthcare provider, we do hope that the information we have included will expand on his or her explanations and advice.

Blood clotting is a normal, protective response to blood vessel injury. Deep vein thrombosis and pulmonary embolism are the result of abnormal blood clotting. The blood clotting process is difficult to understand, even for medical professionals, so the first section of the book provides basic information and terminology that will be helpful in understanding the remainder of the book. The second section describes the symptoms of deep vein thrombosis and pulmonary embolism and explains how the conditions are diagnosed. The third and fourth sections describe the initial and long-term treatment. The circumstances that result in abnormal blood clotting vary from case to case and since there is no single cause of either deep vein thrombosis or pulmonary embolism, the fifth section describes the multiple risk factors for these conditions. The sixth, seventh, and eighth sections address the unique problems that women face. The ninth and tenth sections discuss how other medical conditions, surgery, and trauma affect deep vein thrombosis, pulmonary embolism, and their treatment. The eleventh and twelfth sections answer questions about lifestyle issues such as travel, activity, sports, and recreation. The thirteenth section describes complications that might arise and the fourteenth answers questions about how recurrent clots can be prevented. The fifteenth addresses family and genetic issues. The last section provides answers to miscellaneous questions such as "Who treats deep vein thrombosis and pulmonary embolism?", "What does insurance pay for?" and "Where can more information be found?"

In preparing the book, we were inspired by our patients, some of whom contributed to this book:

- Dena Brown, a mother
- Jennifer, a mother
- David James, a retired engineer
- Marvin Creamer, a retired professor and circumnavigator

We are most grateful for their willingness to share their stories.

One of our patients, Marv Nelson, read the entire manuscript and offered important suggestions for improvement.

We are also grateful to:

- Mike Hefron, Client Unit Director at IBM, whose story we first heard at the Surgeon General's Workshop on DVT in Washington, DC, May of 2006, and
- Lori Preston, MBA, Vice President and co-founder of the National Alliance for Thrombosis and Thrombophilia (NATT)

for contributing their stories.

In preparing this book, we were supported by our colleagues. Kristen Nunez, Genetics Counselor, provided information for the section on family and genetic issues. Whitney Howell, Public Relations Specialist for the Duke Medical Center News Office, proofread the manuscript and asked for clarification of medical terms. Karen Baker, Clinical Nurse Specialist, Kathryn Vokaty, Physician Assistant, Michelle Schoonover, Coagulation Pharmacist, and Kim Hodulik, Coagulation Pharmacist, from the Duke Anticoagulation Clinic read the manuscript and provided helpful suggestions. Our colleague Dr. Richard Becker, cardiologist and expert in deep vein thrombosis and pulmonary embolism, graciously agreed to write the Foreword.

In preparing this book we were encouraged by our family members, especially Karen, David, and Marvin. Therefore, we would like to dedicate this book to our patients, our colleagues, our clinic staff, and our family members who all helped to make this book possible.

Andra H. James, MD
Thomas L. Ortel, MD, PhD
Victor F. Tapson, MD

PART ONE

The Basics

What is blood?

What is the purpose of blood vessels?

How and why does blood clot?

More...

1. What is blood?

Blood is a fluid that transports essential substances around the body. It is composed of **proteins,** other molecules, and cells.

The main type of cell in the blood is the **red blood cell.** Red blood cells contain **hemoglobin,** a molecule that has the unique ability to pick up oxygen in areas of the body where the concentration of oxygen is high (the lungs), carry the oxygen to other parts of the body, and release it where the concentration of oxygen is low (the arms, legs, and organs other than the lungs). Oxygen combines with energy sources derived from food to provide "fuel" to individual cells within the tissue of organs and extremities, ensuring that the cells can survive and function. This process produces carbon dioxide, which must then be carried away. Hemoglobin also has the ability to pick up carbon dioxide where the concentration of carbon dioxide is high (the arms, legs, and organs other than the lungs) and release it where the concentration is low (the lungs). In summary, the red blood cells carry oxygen to the cells within the tissues of organs and extremities and carry carbon dioxide away from those locations.

The other types of cells found in blood are white blood cells and **platelets.** White blood cells fight infection. Platelets help prevent blood from leaking out of injured blood vessels.

2. What is the purpose of blood vessels?

The purpose of blood vessels is to carry blood to organs and extremities. Two major types of blood vessels exist: **arteries** and **veins.**

Arteries are thick, muscular vessels that carry blood away from the heart. Within organs and extremities, arteries branch into smaller vessels called arterioles; the arterioles, in turn, branch into capillaries. Capillaries are thin, tiny vessels that allow molecules, fluids, and even some cells to travel in and out of them.

In contrast to the arteries, veins carry blood back to the heart from organs and extremities. Capillaries branch into larger blood vessels called venules; the venules, in turn, branch into veins. Compared to the arteries, the pressure in the veins is very low. Because veins carry blood back to the heart under low pressure and against gravity, they contain valves that open with forward flow of the blood (when the heart contracts) and close to prevent back flow of the blood (when the heart relaxes).

Blood returns from organs and extremities to the right side of the heart through a very large vein called the **vena cava.** The "superior" branch of the vena cava carries blood from the upper part of the body, and the "inferior" branch of the vena cava carries blood from the lower part of the body. The right side of the heart—particularly the right ventricle—then pumps the blood through a very large artery, called the **pulmonary artery,** to the lungs. The pulmonary artery branches into the left pulmonary artery (which carries blood to the left lung) and the right pulmonary artery (which carries blood to the right lung). Inside the lungs, the right and left pulmonary arteries branch into smaller arterioles and even smaller capillaries. Carbon dioxide passes out of the capillaries into the air sacs (alveoli) of the lungs; simultaneously, oxygen passes out of the alveoli into the capillaries. The newly oxygenated blood travels from the capillaries through the venules and pulmonary veins into the left side of the heart, where it is pumped by the left ventricle through a very large artery, called the aorta, to the rest of the body.

3. How and why does blood clot?

Because normal blood flow is necessary to supply oxygen to organs and extremities and to carry carbon dioxide away from these tissues, damage to a blood vessel could jeopardize life-sustaining functions by allowing blood to leak out. All animals, including humans, have an inborn mechanism by which

The Basics

Hemoglobin

The protein molecule in red blood cells that carries oxygen from the lungs to the body's tissues and returns carbon dioxide from the tissues to the lungs. The iron contained in hemoglobin is responsible for the red color of blood.

Platelet

The smallest cell in the blood. Platelets are important for normal blood clotting; they prevent blood from leaking out of an injured blood vessel.

Artery

A vessel through which the blood passes away from the heart and to the various parts of the body.

Vein

A vessel through which blood passes from various organs back to the heart.

Vena cava

A large vein that carries blood from the tissues to the heart, and then on to the lungs to pick up oxygen. The "superior" branch of the vena cava carries blood from the upper part of the body; the "inferior" branch of the vena cava carries blood from the lower part of the body.

Pulmonary artery

The main blood vessel carrying blood from the right side of the heart (right ventricle) into the lungs to pick up oxygen. This large blood vessel divides into smaller and smaller branches deeper into the lung. The pulmonary arteries are where pulmonary emboli migrate to, and block off.

Coagulation

The process of blood clotting.

Endothelium

The lining of a blood vessel. Damage to the endothelium, such as from trauma (or a previous blood clot), makes a patient more susceptible to a blood clot.

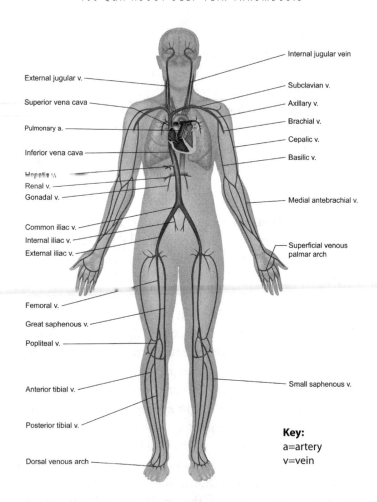

Internal jugular vein
External jugular v.
Superior vena cava
Subclavian v.
Axillary v.
Brachial v.
Pulmonary a.
Cepalic v.
Inferior vena cava
Basilic v.
Hepatic v.
Renal v.
Gonadal v.
Medial antebrachial v.
Common iliac v.
Internal iliac v.
External iliac v.
Superficial venous palmar arch
Femoral v.
Great saphenous v.
Popliteal v.
Anterior tibial v.
Small saphenous v.
Posterior tibial v.
Dorsal venous arch

Key:
a=artery
v=vein

Figure 1   The veins of the body. Superficial leg veins; saphenous; superficial arm veins; cephalic, basilic, and median antebrachial (antecubital)

a possible leak at the site of blood vessel injury is plugged. This mechanism is called blood clotting or **coagulation.**

Blood vessels can be injured in many ways, including minor trauma, serious injury, or surgery. Arteries can also be damaged by certain disease processes such as atherosclerosis, commonly called "hardening of the arteries." Ordinarily, blood vessels are lined by a smooth, slippery surface called the **endothelium.** When blood vessels are injured, the endothelium is damaged and the tissue underneath the endothelium, called the subendothelium, is exposed. The subendothelium is rough and sticky. As a consequence, platelets, which are the cells that prevent blood from leaking out of an injured blood vessel, stick or adhere to the subendothelium where it is exposed. In the process, the platelets change their shape from a disk to a globular shape (like an ameba). During this shape-changing process, certain internal structures or granules are disrupted and release substances that activate the platelets. Activated platelets have receptors on their surfaces that allow them to stick to one another (that is, aggregate). Aggregated platelets form a plug at the site of a possible leak.

This plug remains just a clump of platelets until a mesh or net made of a substance called **fibrin** surrounds these cells. Fibrin is a solid that is formed from **fibrinogen,** a specialized protein or clotting factor that is found in blood. When a blood vessel is injured, the exposed subendothelium causes a protein known as **tissue factor** to be exposed to the blood. The tissue factor sets off a chain reaction, called the coagulation cascade, that activates a whole series of clotting factors. The last step of this chain reaction is the conversion of fibrinogen into fibrin, which forms the mesh that holds the platelets firmly in place. A **clot** (also known as a **thrombus**), therefore, is made up of fibrin, platelets, and other cells, particularly red blood cells that are trapped in the process.

Besides blood vessel injury, two other factors are associated with the development of blood clots: interruption of blood flow (which results in slow, sluggish, or nonexistent blood flow) and an increased tendency within the blood to form clots. The identification of these three factors associated with the development of blood clots is attributed to a famous nineteenth-century German pathologist, Rudolph Virchow (although he did not actually describe them). Blood vessel injury, interruption of blood flow, and the increased tendency toward blood clotting are, therefore, commonly called **Virchow's triad.** Virchow did describe the process whereby some clots detach

All animals, including humans, have an inborn mechanism—called blood clotting (coagulation)—by which a possible leak at the site of blood vessel injury is plugged.

Fibrin

A solid substance formed from fibrinogen, a specialized protein or clotting factor that is found in blood. Fibrin makes a clot more stable (harder to break up). It forms the mesh or net that holds blood platelets firmly in place.

Fibrinogen

A specialized protein or clotting factor that is found in blood. When a blood vessel is injured, another clotting factor, thrombin, is activated and converts fibrinogen to fibrin, which is the mesh or net that holds platelets firmly in place.

Tissue factor

A substance that is released from the blood vessel lining and initiates the clotting reaction.

Clot

A thrombus.

Thrombus

A blood clot.

Virchow's triad

The three basic factors that increase a patient's risk for deep vein thrombosis: (1) stasis (reduced mobility or immobility), (2) injury to a blood vessel, and (3) thrombophilia.

Thrombosis

The pathologic (abnormal) process whereby liquid blood forms a clot within a blood vessel or the heart.

Deep vein thrombosis (DVT)

A condition in which a blood clot forms in the deep veins of the legs, pelvis, or arms. The treatment for DVT includes anticoagulant therapy.

from the subendothelium, travel through larger blood vessels, and become lodged in smaller, remote blood vessels.

Because clots are necessary to prevent blood from leaking out of blood vessels after injury, individuals who have too few platelets, abnormal platelets, platelets that do not function normally, or deficiencies of clotting factors may not form normal clots and may suffer from excessive bleeding. Conversely, when clots form when and where they should not, serious consequences—including death—may occur. For instance, if a clot forms in the arteries supplying the heart (the coronary arteries), blood flow is blocked, the oxygen supply is cut off, and the cells in the heart begin to die, resulting in a myocardial infarction (heart attack). If a clot forms in the arteries supplying the brain, blood flow is blocked, the oxygen supply is cut off, and the cells in the brain begin to die, resulting in a cerebrovascular accident (stroke).

4. What is deep vein thrombosis?

Thrombosis is another word for blood clot. **Deep vein thrombosis (DVT)** refers to the formation of a blood clot in one of the deep veins of the body, usually a vein in the muscle of one of the legs. Two types of thrombosis are distinguished: nonocclusive thrombosis, which does not completely block a vein, and occlusive thrombosis, which does completely block the vein. A blood clot or thrombosis may not be noticed or produce symptoms until it completely occludes a vein.

5. How common is DVT?

The chances of developing DVT are about 1 in 1000 per year, although certain factors greatly increase this risk. Young people are less likely than older people to develop DVT. The cumulative chance of developing DVT over a lifetime ranges from 2 percent to 5 percent. While certain conditions can provoke DVT (such as cancer, surgery, and being confined to bed), this condition may also occur spontaneously. Approximately 20 to 40 percent of people who develop spontaneous DVT have an inherited or **acquired** predisposition to thrombosis or **thrombophilia** (discussed later in this book). An estimated 300,000 first-time cases of DVT occur in the United States every year.

6. Where does DVT occur?

In a study of more than 5000 people with DVT, a blood clot occurred in one leg in 77 percent of cases and in both legs in 12 percent of cases. In 11 percent of cases, the DVT occurred in an arm. In less than 1 percent of individuals, DVT occurred in the veins of the brain, neck, liver, or pelvis or in the inferior vena cava (the very large vein that carries blood back to the heart from the lower part of the body). Thus, while such cases are rare, blood clots may occur in sites other than the legs.

The chances of developing DVT are about 1 in 1000 per year, although certain factors greatly increase this risk. The cumulative chance of developing DVT over a lifetime ranges from 2 percent to 5 percent.

Spontaneous DVT

A clot that forms when there are no obvious risk factors. Twenty to 40 percent of people who develop a spontaneous DVT have an inherited or acquired predisposition to thrombosis or thrombophilia.

Acquired

A condition that is not genetic (inherited) or congenital (present at birth); usually caused by environmental factors and/or other physical conditions.

Dena's story:

When I was 23 years old, I started having severe pains in my stomach—so bad that I couldn't sit up straight. After waiting a few days, and with the pain not subsiding, I visited my family physician and he, unknowingly, gave me something for stomach bloating. Needless to say, that didn't work, and after a couple of days, I went back to him again. He could not find out what was causing my pain, so he sent me directly to a surgeon who specialized in laparoscopic procedures. The surgeon thought that maybe the problem was my appendix, so he decided to go ahead and do an exploratory laparotomy. He removed my appendix, which was normal; tested my lymph nodes for cancer, which were normal; performed tests for sexually transmitted diseases, which were normal; and so on.

When I continued to get worse (my weight went from 119 pounds to 156 pounds in a matter of days), my mother was adamant that I be moved to another hospital. I was transported immediately to another hospital, and a specialist was called in. After seeing the pain I was in and realizing the urgency of the situation, he per-

formed emergency surgery. He found a huge section of my small intestine was dead and removed almost 3 feet of it. He said he was almost positive that a blood clot in my intestines had started this whole ordeal. He asked me if I had taken karate, been kicked in the stomach, or had any trauma to that area, which I hadn't.

The first 48 hours after surgery were critical. The doctors were unsure if I would make it. If I did, they said I might have to wear a colostomy bag. I was very lucky, and all of my organs regained their proper function. After surgery and during my three-week stay in the hospital, I learned that a blood clot had formed in my superior mesenteric vein (a vein in the intestines) and small clots had formed in both common femoral veins (the veins in my groin).

Jennifer's story:

My story started when I was 27 years old and was pregnant. I was nearing my due date when my doctor discovered that my blood pressure was higher than it had been all throughout my pregnancy. My blood pressure had been normal up until this point. It continued to be high, so the doctor sent me to the hospital to do a nonstress test, but everything appeared normal. Once I passed my due date, the doctor recommended that I be induced. I went in early in the morning on a Thursday. My husband and I were very excited. I gave birth later that night to our beautiful and healthy daughter. There were no problems with the delivery, and we both went home three days later.

Monday afternoon, I started having a headache on the back top part of my head. Before I knew it, it was a pounding and I was in a lot of pain. I called my family physician and described the throbbing headache I was having. She told me to go to the emergency room. My husband took me, and when I talked to the doctor there, he said that I might be experiencing an after-effect headache from the epidural that I had received during my labor. Because the records didn't indicate there had been any problems when the epidural was administered, he wasn't sure. He also thought the headache could be due to preeclampsia. The doctor

Thrombophilia

A predisposition to the development of blood clots. It is sometimes referred to as "hypercoagulability." Thrombophilia can be either inherited or acquired during a person's lifetime.

prescribed Tylenol with codeine and advised me to come back in a few days if things didn't get better.

The headaches continued, but the medicine helped to mask them a little bit over the next few days. When I woke up on Friday morning, I was feeling better than I had all week. Because my mother was taking care of our daughter and I was anxious to get back into my regular routine, I went downstairs and started to wash dishes. As I was doing so, my left arm started to go numb. The next thing I knew, it was shaking uncontrollably. This really made me nervous. Thank goodness my mother was there to calm me down and call my family physician. My doctor thought I was having a seizure and sent me to a neurologist, who I saw later that day.

The arm shaking happened again while I was having my appointment with the neurologist. He told me I was having a seizure and wanted to know if I had a history of having seizures or other medical problems. I told him I had never had any seizures or serious medical problems. The neurologist told me he wanted me to have an MRI that evening to rule out a blood clot, a brain tumor, or an aneurysm. I was very nervous and was so glad my husband was with me because I didn't understand why all this was happening. I went to an office downstairs from the neurologist's office to have the MRI done. Once we went back up to his office, he told me nothing showed up on the MRI. Because of the arm seizures, he prescribed an antiseizure medication. He said it could take a few days to take full effect, so I should take it easy.

The next day my husband brought me some lunch as I was resting. All of a sudden, my head turned right around uncontrollably and I went into a full body seizure. I don't remember having the seizure, but afterward I remember my husband on the phone with 911, asking them to send an ambulance. I was so scared. I had never, ever experienced anything like this before.

Shortly after I was taken to the emergency room, I was admitted to the hospital and the neurologist became my main doctor. During my stay, I went through a series of tests to determine a diagnosis. The tests included an angiogram, an electroencephalogram (EEG), a spinal tap, an echocardiogram (a heart ultrasound), and a CT scan. Although the spinal tap showed some "old" blood was in the spine and brain, and the EEG showed some abnormalities, most of the tests came back normal. My doctor didn't know what the problem was, but he thought it could be epilepsy or preeclampsia. The doctor did not discover the clot during all of this testing, but I continued to have symptoms. My headaches occurred daily, and I even lost motor skills on the left side of my body. I experienced numbness in my arms and legs on my left side, and I had tingling above my lips. I did have a couple of seizures during my stay, but the seizures subsided as I continued to take the medication. After about two weeks, the doctor let me go home, even though I continued to have headaches and was not feeling well. There was still no diagnosis.

For the next three days, I lay listless in my bed with constant pain in my head and no appetite. No over-the-counter medicine helped. My husband called the doctor each day. Because my condition was getting worse, on the third day, the doctor ordered another MRI. This time, a dye was injected into a vein that helps "light up" the veins in the brain. That is when they discovered that I had a blood clot in a vein in my brain.

PART TWO

Diagnosis and Symptoms

What are the symptoms of DVT?

What is the difference between DVT and superficial vein thrombosis or superficial thrombophlebitis?

How is DVT diagnosed?

More . . .

7. What are the symptoms of DVT?

The classic symptoms of DVT are pain, swelling, tenderness to the touch along the course of the vein, redness, or even bluish discoloration of the affected arm or leg.

DVT usually occurs in a leg or, less often, in an arm. Sometimes a clot is small or only partially obstructs a blood vessel, and there are no symptoms. The classic symptoms, however, are pain, swelling, tenderness to the touch along the course of the vein, redness, or, in some cases, even bluish discoloration of the affected arm or leg. It is possible to have these symptoms without having DVT. In fact, a diagnosis of DVT is confirmed in only 25 percent of such cases. Other conditions that can cause the same or similar symptoms include an infection, a bruised muscle, or the rupture of one of the fluid sacs or "bursa" that cushion the tissue around the knee. The latter condition is called a ruptured Baker's cyst.

Marvin's story:

I have had four episodes of DVT or pulmonary embolism (PE). In retrospect, the first episode, which occurred in my right leg, was never diagnosed and eventually got better on its own.

The second episode, which was the first recognized episode, began with a severe pain in the left calf muscle. It felt much like a cramp but did not yield to any kind of manipulation. The onset came 10 days after a gastroenterologist had removed a polyp from my colon. Wondering if there might be a connection, I asked the gastroenterologist. He thought not, but suggested I see my family physician. Because my family doctor had died recently, I had to see a doctor who was not known to me—a general practitioner. When I visited him, he bent the toes of my left foot back. Because I didn't wince, the doctor concluded the pain in my calf was not a clot but merely inflammation of the gastrocnemius muscle (a muscle in the calf), for which he prescribed a regimen of butazoladin (a nonsteroidal anti-inflammatory drug that is no longer on the market). It did not relieve the symptoms or alter the condition.

Nonetheless, because I had been reassured that my pain was only muscle inflammation, I kept my commitments, which included an appearance on a television show. I drove 120 miles to New York City, stayed overnight, appeared for the taping, and drove home the next day. All the while, the severe pain remained untouched by pain relievers. I checked back with the gastroenterologist, and he asked me to come in immediately for an emergency visit. When he saw the swollen and painful leg, he ordered a gurney and had me transferred to the hospital, where I spent five days for the initial treatment of a DVT.

8. What is the difference between DVT and superficial vein thrombosis or superficial thrombophlebitis?

Superficial vein thrombosis is also called **superficial thrombophlebitis.** Symptoms include pain, swelling, and redness along the course of a superficial vein. While DVT occurs in a deep vein, a superficial vein thrombosis occurs in a superficial vein. Superficial veins, which are sometimes visible on the arms or legs, collect blood underneath the surface of the skin. They are not deep. They do not carry blood directly back to the heart, but instead transfer blood to the deep veins through small communicating veins.

Because superficial veins do not carry blood directly back to the heart, the consequences of a superficial vein thrombosis are not the same as those associated with DVT. Even if the clot or a piece of the clot breaks free, it cannot fit through the small communicating veins and cannot travel to the heart and wedge itself into one of the pulmonary arteries or its branches, resulting in a pulmonary embolism (PE). (See Question 10.) Therefore, superficial vein thrombosis does not necessarily require treatment with **anticoagulation,** unlike DVT and PE. Treatment usually consists of heat; nonsteroidal anti-inflammatory drugs, such as ibuprofen (Motrin®, Advil®, Nuprin®) or naproxen (Aleve®, Orudis KT); **fitted elastic compression stockings;** and elevation of the affected extremity. Symptoms usually disappear in two to six weeks. Sometimes anticoagulation is used to help alleviate

Superficial thrombophlebitis

A blood clot or clots that form in the veins nearer to the surface.

Anticoagulation

A general term for a treatment that interferes with the ability of the blood to form a normal blood clot. Anticoagulant medicines include heparin and warfarin, and are sometimes referred to as "blood thinners."

Fitted elastic compression stockings

Elastic stockings, which ideally exert a pressure of at least 30 to 40 mm Hg at the ankle with less pressure at the knee. Fitted elastic compression stockings provide counter-pressure to veins and help return fluid that has leaked out of them back into the circulation.

the symptoms. If the condition worsens or does not improve, DVT should be considered.

9. How is DVT diagnosed?

In the diagnosis of DVT, the physician considers the patient's specific risk factors, the patient's symptoms, the physical examination, other possible explanations for the symptoms, and the results of objective tests, such as some method of imaging (that is, seeing) the clot.

Duplex Ultrasound

The first method that is usually performed in an attempt to image the clot is **ultrasound**—specifically, duplex ultrasound. "Duplex" refers to the two parts of the process.

Ultrasound

A test used to identify a number of medical conditions. When DVT is suspected, the inability to compress the leg veins with the ultrasound device indicates the presence of DVT. Abnormal blood flow can also be demonstrated when DVT is present.

In the first part of the process, brightness modulation ultrasound (also known as B-mode ultrasound) is used to obtain an image or picture. The ultrasound machine creates high-energy sound waves (ultrasound) that are bounced off internal tissues and make echoes. The patterns of these echoes form an image, which is then shown on the screen of the machine. While imaging the deep veins of the leg, the sonographer (the person who operates the ultrasound machine) tries to collapse or compress the veins. If a vein cannot be compressed because a clot prevents the vein from collapsing, a DVT diagnosis is made. The ability to completely flatten a vein with compression is the most useful way to be certain that a clot is not present.

In the second part of the duplex ultrasound process, Doppler ultrasound is used to detect abnormalities of blood flow. Sound waves are bounced off the blood within a vein. Flowing blood changes the sound waves by the "Doppler effect." The ultrasound machine can detect these changes and determine whether blood within a vein is flowing normally. Absence of blood flow confirms the diagnosis of DVT.

Duplex ultrasound successfully identifies 95 percent of deep vein thromboses that occur in the large veins above the knee.

The ability of duplex ultrasound to detect DVT in the large veins above the knee is so good that when the test is positive, no further testing is necessary and treatment may be started. Conversely, if the test is negative, the chance that there is a DVT is so small that treatment may safely be withheld.

This technique is not as good at detecting DVT that occurs below the knee or in the calf veins, however. Duplex ultrasound successfully identifies only 60 to 70 percent of calf vein thromboses. Even when such a diagnosis is made, it is correct only 60 to 70 percent of the time. While calf vein thromboses account for 20 percent of all DVT cases, only one in five these thromboses ever grows in the first week or two after it is initially suspected. Also, calf vein thromboses are less likely to break free and travel to the lung or "embolize." Therefore, if the ultrasound is negative, even though a DVT may be present in a calf vein, treatment may be withheld and the ultrasound repeated in five to seven days if the symptoms persist. Calf vein thrombosis may be treated like superficial thrombophlebitis. Most physicians prescribe **anticoagulants** in such cases, however, because a DVT in a calf vein can lead to a larger, more proximal DVT that can break off and migrate to the lung.

Duplex Ultrasound in Recurrent DVT

Abnormalities of the veins are common after DVT, making it difficult to diagnose a recurrent clot. For instance, half of the time the results of the duplex ultrasound remain abnormal one year after the first episode of DVT. Consequently, if duplex ultrasound is being performed to determine whether a new clot has developed, lack of compression or absence of blood flow does not prove the existence of a new clot unless a new segment of the vein or a different vein is involved.

Venography and Magnetic Resonance Imaging

If the ultrasound is negative, yet the patient's symptoms are severe or a DVT is strongly suspected, the next step is either a venogram (venography) or **magnetic resonance imaging**

Magnetic resonance imaging (MRI)

A test that images clots in the body. While MRI does a better job of imaging the veins in the pelvis, abdomen, and chest than ultrasound does, ultrasound for the legs is usually adequate (and is cheaper). Neither test exposes a patient to radiation.

(MRI). Sometimes the ultrasound is negative because there is a clot in a vein in the pelvis, hidden from the ultrasound. Although isolated pelvic vein thrombosis is uncommon, it can occur in women who are pregnant or who have recently delivered a baby, in people who have had pelvic cancer, or in people who have had recent pelvic surgery.

Until recently, venography using x-rays was used to diagnose DVT. During venography, contrast dye (usually an iodine dye), which helps blood vessels show up clearly on x-ray, was injected into a vein in the foot. A series of x-rays of the veins was then taken, looking for blockages. Today, the use of x-ray venography has been almost entirely replaced by the use of ultrasound and magnetic resonance (MR) venography, because x-ray venography is "invasive" and can be painful. The MR machine uses pulses of radio-frequency waves to cause hydrogen atoms to line up within tissues. When the pulse stops, the hydrogen atoms return to their natural state. In the process, they give off a signal that the machine converts into an image. Different tissues give off different signals. Because clots give off different signals than flowing blood, MR can be used to detect a thrombosis.

MR venography does a better job of imaging the veins in the pelvis, abdomen, and chest than ultrasound does. Because it does not require compression, this technology can be used to detect clots in limbs inside of plaster casts. Overall, MR may be superior to ultrasound, but it is a much more involved test and costs much more than ultrasound.

Lyse or lysis

To lyse a clot is to dissolve or destroy a clot. Lysis is the process whereby a clot is dissolved or destroyed. This process can occur naturally over time or can be accomplished by powerful, clot-busting drugs (thrombolytics).

D-Dimer Test

After a blood clot starts to form, another series of reactions normally begins to dissolve (that is, **lyse**) the clot. Fibrin, which forms the mesh that holds the platelets firmly in place within a clot, is a solid that is formed from fibrinogen, a specialized protein (clotting factor) found in blood. (See Question 3.) These fibrinogen molecules are strung together end-to-end and cross-linked within fibrin.

During the lysis process, fibrin is broken down or degraded by an enzyme called plasmin. Plasmin cuts the strands of fibrin on either side of what were the ends of the fibrinogen molecules. These ends are called "D" units. A *dimer* is a pair, so the **D-dimer** is a fragment of cross-linked fibrin that consists of two "D" units. D-dimers can be present in a variety of conditions, including the formation of a blood clot. While the presence of D-dimers does not guarantee that a blood clot is present, it is a clue that the clotting process has begun. If D-dimers are absent, however, it is very unlikely that a blood clot has begun to form. For that reason, a blood test for D-dimers is often performed to ensure that a blood clot is absent.

A number of tests for D-dimers exist. If such a test is intended to prove that a blood clot is absent, then the test should be a sensitive one (one that will detect D-dimers whenever they are present). Also, the test should be interpreted in the context of an individual's situation.

Recent research suggests that testing for D-dimers when discontinuation of **warfarin** therapy is being considered may help identify the best time to stop the warfarin. If the D-dimer test is normal, it might suggest that it is safe to stop anticoagulation and that the patient's risk for experiencing a recurrent clot may be lower. More research is being done in this area.

10. What are the consequences of DVT?

After a blood clot starts to form, another series of reactions almost immediately begins to dissolve (lyse) the clot. The purpose of this process is to confine the clot to the injured area of the blood vessel, limit the size of the clot, and prevent it from growing too large. Sometimes DVT can be completely dissolved or lysed by the body's own natural processes. Even under these circumstances, however, the clot is likely to cause permanent damage to the vein and its valves. In fact, 5 to 30 percent of individuals who experience DVT develop a second or recurrent DVT within five years of the first episode.

While the presence of D-dimers does not guarantee that a blood clot is present, it is a clue that the clotting process has begun. If D-dimers are absent, it is very unlikely that a blood clot has begun to form.

D-dimer

A breakdown product of fibrin, which is present in a blood clot. D-dimers are not generally present in the blood unless a clot has begun to form, although the presence of D-dimers does not guarantee that a clot is present. If D-dimers are absent, it is very unlikely that a blood clot has begun to form.

Warfarin

A medicine given by mouth that interferes with blood clotting and is generally used for the prevention or treatment of blood clots. It is often referred to as a "blood thinner."

As many as 600,000 Americans are hospitalized each year for DVT and its primary complication, PE. In the United States, DVT and PE account for as many as 300,000 deaths per year.

Sometimes, a clot serves as a surface on which another clot forms, so that the clot continues to grow. As it increases in size, blood flow may be completely blocked within a vein. The clot may even extend into the larger vein to which the present vein is connected. In this case, circulation to a leg, arm, or other organ may be so impaired that the limb, organ, or person's life may be threatened.

In one of every five cases, the clot (or a piece of it) breaks free and travels through progressively larger veins, through the vena cava, and through the right side of the heart, and then wedges into one of the pulmonary arteries or its branches, resulting in **pulmonary embolism (PE)**. As many as 600,000 Americans are hospitalized each year for DVT and its primary complication, PE. In the United States, DVT and PE account for as many as 300,000 deaths per year.

Three to four percent of all patients who experience PE suffer from chronic (persistent) obstruction of blood flow through the lungs—a condition known as **chronic thromboembolic pulmonary hypertension (CTEPH)**. The obstruction of this blood flow increases the blood pressure in the pulmonary arteries, which carry blood from the right side of the heart to the lungs. CTEPH therefore strains the right side of the heart, causing symptoms of heart failure including shortness of breath. (See Questions 80 and 81.)

11. What is post-phlebitic or post-thrombotic syndrome?

Approximately 30 percent of people who experience DVT develop chronic symptoms as a consequence of permanent injury to veins and their valves. These symptoms may not emerge right away. In fact, after one to two years, only 10 to 20 percent of people experience these symptoms; after five years, however, 20 to 30 percent do.

Chronic symptoms include swelling, pain, and discoloration of the skin. A rusty discoloration of the skin, caused by iron

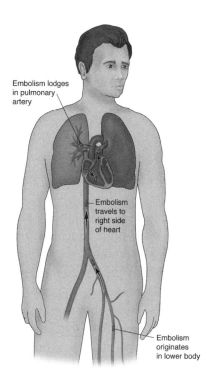

Embolism lodges in pulmonary artery

Embolism travels to right side of heart

Embolism originates in lower body

Figure 2   Pulmonary Embolism. A pulmonary embolism is a blood clot that forms in a vein, breaks off, circulates through the venous system, and moves through the right side of the heart into the pulmonary artery. It can become lodged and significantly obstruct blood flow.

deposits from old blood, is often the first sign, followed by chronic swelling. In severe cases, the skin can break down, allowing an **ulcer** (open sore) to form. After one year, only 2 to 3 percent of people develop these ulcers; by contrast, after five years, as many as 10 to 20 percent may suffer from such an ulcer on the legs. Not surprisingly, **post-phlebitic (post-thrombotic) syndrome** is more likely to develop after DVT that was associated with symptoms as opposed to a DVT that was diagnosed by imaging alone. (See Questions 80 and 81.)

12. What is pulmonary embolism?

The pulmonary embolism (PE) process was first described by Rudolph Virchow, the famous nineteenth-century German pathologist who called the traveling clots *embolia*. The terms

Chronic thromboembolic pulmonary hypertension (CTEPH)

High blood pressure in the lungs that occurs in a small percentage of patients who have had pulmonary embolism. The most common symptom is shortness of breath. This problem usually progresses but may be cured with surgery.

Ulcer

A chronic (long-standing) open sore.

Post-phlebitic (post-thrombotic) syndrome

Long-term, recurring leg symptoms that affect some patients as a result of permanent injury to veins and their valves from DVT.

19

"embolus" (plural: emboli) and "embolism" are still used to describe a clot or part of a clot that has formed in one site and traveled to another part of the body. When a clot wedges itself in one of the pulmonary arteries or its branches, it is called PE.

A very large PE can block the entire trunk of the pulmonary artery (before it branches into the right and left pulmonary arteries) and cause death instantly. Pulmonary emboli that are not quite so large may block an entire right or left pulmonary artery, stopping the blood flow to an entire lung and—especially if the person already has lung or heart disease—causing death. Smaller emboli may block smaller branches of the pulmonary artery with varying consequences. When the blood supply to a small "end-artery" at the edge of the lung is blocked, oxygen to that part of the lung is cut off, and the cells in that part of the lung begin to die, resulting in **pulmonary infarction** (that is, death of lung tissue). When blood flow is blocked within a larger branch of the pulmonary artery, the normal exchange of oxygen for carbon dioxide does not take place and the entire body is affected. Pulmonary infarctions usually result from smaller clots and are unlikely to be fatal.

The likelihood of death from PE depends largely on the size of the PE. If the main pulmonary artery is completely blocked, the right ventricle (the chamber of the heart that pumps blood into the lungs) cannot get the blood into the lungs; this "right ventricular failure" then leads to death from PE. The age and health of the affected individual are also critical factors. When the person already has lung or heart disease, PE may have a more dramatic impact. While the death rate from PE may be as high as 25 percent in sick, hospitalized patients, the death rate in young healthy individuals is closer to 1 percent.

Pulmonary infarction

The death of a small area of lung resulting from pulmonary embolism that occurs in a small, dead-end pulmonary artery. Pulmonary infarction often causes pain in the chest or back.

The likelihood of death from PE depends largely on the size of the PE.

13. What are the symptoms of PE?

While the vast majority of pulmonary emboli are believed to originate in the deep veins of the body, fewer than 30 percent of individuals who experience PE have symptoms of DVT. Instead, the most common symptoms are shortness of breath and chest pain. In the Prospective Investigation of Pulmonary Embolism Diagnosis (PIOPED) study, a large study conducted by the National Heart Lung and Blood Institute of the National Institute of Health, 73 percent of patients with PE experienced shortness of breath, 66 percent experienced chest pain, 37 percent experienced cough, and 13 percent coughed up blood. During physical examination, 70 percent had rapid breathing and 30 percent had a rapid heart rate. When doctors listened to the study participants with a stethoscope, half had abnormal sounds in their lungs and one fourth had abnormal sounds in their hearts. Fourteen percent had a fever.

The most common symptoms of PE are shortness of breath and chest pain, but in some cases, PE may occur very suddenly, without any warning.

In some cases, PE may occur very suddenly, without any warning. The symptoms of PE, when noted, are also very nonspecific. For example, shortness of breath and chest pain may occur with pneumonia, bronchitis, or other lung or heart problems. Chest pain may be caused by a number of problems, including muscle strain, heart problems, lung infections, stomach problems such as acid reflux or hiatal hernia, or even anxiety. Whenever a patient has symptoms such as shortness of breath or chest pain, especially when the person has other risk factors for DVT (such as recent surgery, admission to the hospital for a medical disease, or recent immobility), PE should be considered as a possibility.

David's story:

At age 35, I was into my ninth year as an electrical engineer. My involvement with the medical profession was brief and infrequent. I had a broken arm at age 4, all the vaccinations required to go to school, the usual childhood diseases (measles, mumps, chickenpox, and so on), a couple of lacerations that needed stitches, a few ear infections, a bout with hepatitis while in college—and that was about it. In other words, I was healthy.

One morning, I arrived at the plant, climbed the stairs two at a time (as I usually did to go to my office and lab on the second floor), and found myself at the top of the stairs gasping for breath and almost passing out. Because I had never experienced anything like this before, I was frightened, but not enough to seek immediate medical attention. I waited. In 30 minutes, I was breathing normally. I did call the office of the family doctor who saw our children. The receptionist asked me what I needed and I told her I needed a physical exam. She gave me an appointment for three weeks hence.

Meanwhile, I tried some self-diagnosis. I thought that I would try to get the episode to reoccur by running on the treadmill. Fortunately, it didn't reoccur, but over the next two weeks, I started to feel more tired by the end of the day. In the third week after the episode, I was feeling really awful, so my wife called the doctor, and he came to our house that night. His diagnosis was a viral infection. His advice was to tough it out.

Two days later, I was so weak that I had to crawl to get to the toilet. My wife called the doctor again, who again came to the house. He still thought it was a viral infection, but because I was scheduled for my physical exam the next day, he told me that when I came into the office, I should get, among other things, a chest x-ray. The chest x-ray revealed a case of pneumonia. I was so sick that the doctor's partner admitted me to the hospital to start intravenous (IV) antibiotics.

On the second night in the hospital, I got up to go to the toilet and collapsed on the floor gasping for breath. The staff put me back in bed, and in about 30 minutes I wasn't short of breath anymore. In the morning, the doctor's partner ordered a CT scan, which revealed several blood clots in my lungs. I was immediately taken to the intensive care unit and started on IV heparin. Three weeks later, I was out of the hospital, pneumonia under control, arterial blood gases normal, and taking Coumadin®. Six months later, I was told to stop the Coumadin®, start an exercise program, and take an aspirin a day. I did this for 30 years without another episode.

Two years ago, I contracted a case of Rocky Mountain spotted fever from a tick bite. I spent almost a week in bed with high fevers. A couple of nights later, I awakened with severe cramps in my lower ribcage. Hoping the problem would go away, I didn't wake my wife. I felt better the next morning. When I finally told my wife about the episode, she asked me if I thought it could be a PE. I said "no," because the PE 30 years earlier was accompanied by acute shortness of breath, and this episode was not.

Three days later, we started a 10-day vacation that included several airplane rides, including a round trip between New York City and Rome. Upon return from vacation, I resumed my customary exercise on the treadmill. I noticed that my stamina was basically half of what it had been a month before. I chalked it up to a month away from the gym, but after two weeks with no improvement, I contacted my internist, who scheduled me for a stress test the next day.

That next morning, I noticed that I got winded climbing the stairs in our house. Just walking outside to get the paper made me feel light-headed. I was concerned enough to inform my wife, who was getting ready for work. Her approach was to head for the emergency room.

The diagnosis was a PE! I had been fooled. From my experience 30 years ago, I thought I knew what a PE felt like, but apparently different episodes can be accompanied by different symptoms. The symptoms I had 32 years ago were acute shortness of breath and loss of stamina. The symptoms I had 2 years ago were cramps in the lower ribcage and gradual loss of stamina, but no shortness of breath. By the time I reached the emergency room, an echocardiogram revealed that the right side of my heart was beginning to fail. I was immediately started on Lovenox® and admitted to the intensive care unit for tissue plasminogen activator (TPA) to help dissolve the clot. Now, I take Coumadin® every day, but I am lucky to be alive.

14. How is PE diagnosed?

A number of different things may alert the physician that PE may be present (See Question 13). When it is suspected, testing must be considered.

Pulse Oximetry

Often, the first test performed when PE is suspected is a blood oxygen level. The simplest way to measure the blood oxygen level is with a pulse oximeter. **Pulse oximetry** is a noninvasive way (does not involve a blood draw or needle stick) to monitor the percentage of hemoglobin that is saturated with oxygen. Hemoglobin is the unique molecule in red blood cells that has the ability to carry oxygen. The pulse oximeter consists of a probe or sensor plus a computer. The probe, which looks like a padded clothespin, is placed on a relatively thin part of a person's body, such as a finger or earlobe. Both red and infrared light are then transmitted through the tissue by the probe. Based on the absorption of the red and infrared light caused by the difference in color between hemoglobin that is saturated with oxygen (red) and unsaturated hemoglobin (blue), the computer can estimate the proportion of hemoglobin that is oxygenated. The pulse oximeter then displays this result as a percentage. A blood oxygen saturation level less than 95 percent is abnormal. It may be explained by a lung or heart problem already present, such as emphysema or pneumonia, or by PE (or both).

Arterial Blood Gas

A more precise measurement of blood oxygen level is obtained from a sample taken directly from an artery with a needle or a thin tube (catheter). An **arterial blood gas (ABG)** measures the levels of both oxygen and carbon dioxide in the blood to determine how well the lungs are working. While most

Pulse oximetry

A noninvasive (no blood needed!) method of monitoring the percentage of hemoglobin that is saturated with oxygen. A low saturation may be caused by a number of lung or heart diseases, including pulmonary embolism.

Arterial blood gas (ABG)

A technique used primarily to measure the oxygen level of blood with precision. It is obtained from a sample taken directly from an artery with a needle or a thin tube (catheter).

blood tests are performed on samples taken from a vein, an ABG is performed on a sample taken from an artery. In most cases, the artery in the wrist is used for this purpose, but other arteries may be used. The levels of blood gases are measured as partial pressures in units of millimeters of mercury (mm Hg). A partial pressure of oxygen less than 80 mm Hg is abnormal.

Chest X-Ray

A chest x-ray cannot prove that PE is present or absent because clots do not show up on x-ray. Nevertheless, a chest x-ray is a useful test in the evaluation for PE because it can find other diseases, such as pneumonia or fluid in the lungs, that may explain a person's symptoms. Occasionally, when pulmonary infarction occurs, the x-ray may suggest this diagnosis, although more testing is necessary to prove it with certainty. A normal or negative chest x-ray with a low, otherwise unexplained blood oxygen level, however, raises the suspicion for PE.

Ventilation-Perfusion Scan (VQ Scan)

A **VQ lung scan** may be a useful test to determine whether a person has experienced PE. This test evaluates both air flow (V = ventilation) and blood flow (Q = perfusion) in the lungs. About one hour before the test, a slightly radioactive version of the mineral technetium mixed with liquid protein is administered through a vein to identify areas of the lung that may have reduced blood flow. Multiple images are taken from different angles, using a special camera that detects radioactivity. For half of the images, the person breathes from a tube that contains a mixture of air, oxygen, and a slightly radioactive version of the gas xenon, which reveals air flow in different parts of the lung. For the other half of the images, the camera tracks the technetium, which reveals blood flow in different parts of the lung. PE is suspected in areas of the lung that have significant "mismatches"—that is, good air flow but poor blood flow.

VQ lung scan

A test to evaluate both air flow (V = ventilation) and blood flow (Q = perfusion) in the lungs to determine whether a person has experienced a pulmonary embolism.

Except for the minor discomfort from having an intravenous catheter placed, a VQ lung scan is painless and usually takes less than an hour. The exposure to radioactivity from the test is very minor and results in no side effects or complications.

A radiologist interprets the images from the VQ lung scan and decides whether the probability of a PE is high, low, or intermediate. If the probability is high, the diagnosis is made. If the probability is low or intermediate (that is, nondiagnostic), or if the VQ scan cannot be interpreted clearly, other testing must be considered. Even when PE is ultimately proven to be present, the VQ scan may be nondiagnostic. If clinical suspicion is low and the VQ scan reveals a low probability of PE, generally no further testing is needed. A normal VQ scan means PE is not present.

Spiral Computed Tomography of the Chest

An alternative to the VQ scan is a spiral computed tomography (CT) of the chest. A spiral CT of the chest uses special equipment to obtain multiple cross-sectional x-ray images of the organs and tissues of the chest. CT produces images that are far more detailed than those available with a conventional x-ray. Many different types of tissues—including the lungs, heart, bones, soft tissues, muscles, and blood vessels—can be seen. When PE is suspected, contrast dye (usually iodine dye) is administered through a vein to make the blood vessels stand out.

During the spiral CT, radiation is emitted from a rotating tube. Different tissues absorb this radiation differently. During each rotation, approximately 1,000 images are recorded, which a computer then reassembles to produce a detailed image of the interior of the chest. The x-ray rotates as the patient passes through the CT scanner in a spiral path—hence the term "spiral" CT. The amount of radiation exposure is relatively low, and the procedure is not invasive.

Pulmonary Angiogram

If the VQ scan interpretation is low, intermediate, or uncertain probability of PE, or if the spiral CT is normal yet the symptoms are still suspicious, then the definitive test is a **pulmonary angiogram.** An angiogram is an invasive test that uses x-rays to reveal blockages or other abnormalities within the veins or arteries. Contrast dye (usually iodine dye) helps blood vessels show up clearly on x-rays. During an angiogram, contrast dye is injected into a blood vessel, and its path is tracked by a series of x-rays.

Pulmonary angiogram

The most definitive test to diagnose PE. Pulmonary angiogram is an "invasive" test, requiring injection of a dye through a catheter (IV line) into the body. Because newer tests such as CT scanning are now available, pulmonary angiography is rarely needed today.

A pulmonary angiogram examines the arteries that carry blood from the heart to the lungs and is performed to see if PE is present. Using x-rays in real-time (fluoroscopy), the radiologist inserts a catheter into a vein and advances it until it reaches the vena cava (the very large vein that carries blood to the heart). Next, the radiologist advances the catheter still farther into the right side of the heart and finally into the pulmonary artery, the large artery that carries blood to the lungs. The radiologist directs the tip of the catheter into the different branches of the right and left pulmonary arteries and injects the contrast dye, which illuminates the arteries on x-ray. If PE is present, it will show up as a blockage.

Risks associated with a pulmonary angiogram include the possibility of damage caused by the catheter, bleeding, and an allergic reaction to the contrast dye. The amount of radiation from the x-rays is too small to cause any harm.

Echocardiogram

An echocardiogram is an ultrasound of the heart. Doppler ultrasound, B-mode ultrasound, and M-mode ultrasound (a rapid sequence of B-mode images that allows motion to be visualized) are combined to give information about the size of the heart, the function of the valves, and the strength of the heart muscle. (Duplex ultrasound is discussed in more detail in Question 9.) The echocardiogram can spot areas of the heart that are not working well. When patients with a PE have an echocardiogram, approximately 40 percent will be found to have abnormalities of the right side of the heart, particularly the right ventricle. While an echocardiogram is not actually used to diagnose a PE, it can identify strain on the right side of the heart caused by a large PE as well as certain heart problems that may imitate a PE.

PART THREE

Initial Treatment

What are the goals of treatment of DVT?

What is the initial treatment of DVT?

What is heparin?

More . . .

15. What are the goals of treatment of DVT?

The goals of treatment of DVT are fourfold: (1) to prevent a DVT from growing in size, (2) to prevent a DVT from recurring, (3) to prevent PE from developing, and (4) to minimize complications.

16. What is the initial treatment of DVT?

The initial treatment of both DVT and PE is anticoagulation. Anticoagulants, commonly referred to as "blood thinners," do not actually thin blood. Instead, they block the action of various clotting factors and prevent blood clots from growing. In this way, they allow the body's own natural processes to destroy clots over time.

Low-molecular-weight heparin (LMWH)

Chemically cut or cleaved heparin. LMWH lasts longer, must be monitored differently, and generally has fewer side effects than standard heparin.

In the last 10 years, the anticoagulants that have been used for the initial treatment of DVT and PE have changed somewhat. Rather than initial treatment with standard or "unfractionated" heparin, patients are often started on **low-molecular-weight heparin (LMWH)**. Studies have shown that LMWH is at least as effective as standard heparin, but is more convenient to use and has fewer side effects. Compared to standard heparin, LMWH has a longer duration of action, so it requires only daily or twice-daily injections. LMWH also does not have to be directly administered into a vein (unlike standard heparin), but rather can be injected underneath the skin or subcutaneously, usually underneath the skin of the abdomen. Neither heparin nor LMWH can be given by mouth, however. Because LMWH is usually dispensed in prepared (already drawn-up) syringes, many patients with DVT do not require admission to the hospital for treatment. They (or another family member) can be taught how to give themselves injections of LMWH and, therefore, can avoid a hospital stay.

Three LMWHs have been approved by the U.S. Food and Drug Administration (FDA) for the prevention of DVT and PE: dalteparin (Fragmin®), tinzaparin (Innohep®), and enoxaparin (Lovenox®). Only two of these medications, tinzaparin and enoxaparin, have been approved for the treatment of DVT and PE.

Fondaparinux (Arixtra®) is a new type of anticoagulant that has been used for the prevention of DVT and PE and has recently been approved by the FDA for the treatment of DVT and PE. Like LMWH, it cannot be given by mouth or infused intravenously, but it can be given subcutaneously. Fondaparinux has an even longer duration of action than LMWH and requires only once-daily injections.

17. What is heparin?

Heparin is a naturally occurring anticoagulant. While Dr. Jay McLean is often given credit for discovering heparin while he was a medical student, it was his mentor and laboratory director at Johns Hopkins University, Dr. William Howell, and another medical student, Emmett Holt, who first isolated this natural anticoagulant from dog liver in the 1920s and coined the term "heparin." Later in the same decade, at the University of Toronto, heparin was first purified in sufficient quantities from beef liver, and later beef lungs and intestines, to treat humans. Heparin is still derived mainly from beef and sometimes pork sources. It cannot be taken by mouth, but must be administered directly into a vein or injected underneath the skin.

18. How does heparin work?

During the formation of a clot, factor X and factor V work together to convert **prothrombin** (factor II) to **thrombin.** Thrombin is the clotting factor that converts fibrinogen to fibrin. Fibrin is the mesh that holds platelets firmly in place during the formation of a clot. (See Question 3.) Antithrombin is a natural blood thinner that blocks the conversion of factor X to its active form, factor Xa, and also blocks the

Heparin

An anticoagulant medicine ("blood thinner") that is routinely prescribed for the treatment of clotting disorders, including treatment of clots in the coronary arteries (causing heart attack), clots in the blood vessels of the brain (leading to stroke), clots that occur in leg veins (deep vein thrombosis), and clots that obstruct blood flow to the lungs (pulmonary emboli).

Prothrombin

A protein in the blood that is essential for the formation of a blood clot. The active form of prothrombin is called thrombin.

Thrombin

The clotting factor that converts fibrinogen to fibrin.

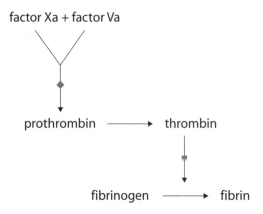

factor Xa + factor Va

prothrombin ⟶ thrombin

fibrinogen ⟶ fibrin

Figure 3   The coagulation cascade.

conversion of prothrombin to thrombin, thereby preventing the conversion of fibrinogen to fibrin. Heparin works by multiplying the action of antithrombin by 1,000-fold.

19. What is the difference between heparin and low-molecular-weight heparin?

Low-molecular-weight heparin (LMWH) is made from standard or "unfractionated" heparin that has been chemically cut or cleaved. Consequently, these partial heparin molecules are of lower weight and behave differently than molecules of standard heparin. They have relatively more activity against factor Xa and relatively less activity against prothrombin. LMWH has a longer duration of action than standard heparin and is less likely to result in bruising, bleeding, or a decrease in the number of platelets (a rare complication that develops in some patients who are treated with heparin). Because LMWH behaves differently from standard heparin, when it is monitored, different tests than those for standard heparin must be used.

20. How is the dose of heparin or LMWH determined?

When LMWH is used to treat DVT or PE, the amount of enoxaparin or tinzaparin prescribed is based on the patient's weight. The initial dose of enoxaparin used to treat DVT or PE is 1 milligram of drug per kilogram of body weight (1 kilogram = 2.2 pounds) given every 12 hours. The initial dose of tinzaparin used to treat DVT or PE is 175 international units (IU) of anti-factor Xa activity per kilogram of body weight given every 12 hours. (Tinzaparin doses are not calculated in milligrams.) These doses of enoxaparin and tinzaparin are considered "full doses." Lower doses are used to prevent DVT or PE.

One advantage of LMWH over standard heparin is that when full doses of LMWH are used to treat DVT or PE, blood levels do not usually have to be monitored. Monitoring is recommended in patients who have certain other conditions such as morbid obesity, kidney disease, or pregnancy. When monitored, LMWH levels are checked with a blood test that measures the medication's activity against clotting factor Xa. Standard heparin is monitored with a different blood test, the activated partial thromboplastin time.

21. What is the activated partial thromboplastin time?

The **activated partial thromboplastin time (aPTT)** test is a blood test that measures the length of time (in seconds) that it takes for clotting to occur when certain substances are added to the liquid portion of blood in a test tube. A normal result requires normal levels of clotting factors VIII, IX, XI, and XII; pre-kallikrein and high-molecular-weight kininogen; and factors V and X, prothrombin, and fibrinogen. The aPTT is used not only to detect clotting factor deficiencies, but also used to monitor heparin's effectiveness.

22. How does fondaparinux work?

Fondaparinux (Arixtra®) differs from standard heparin and LMWH in several ways. In particular, it does not come from animal sources. Instead, this drug is a synthetic version of the active site of the heparin molecule and is an even smaller mol-

Activated partial thromboplastin time (aPTT)

A blood test that measures the length of time (in seconds) that it takes for clotting to occur when certain substances are added to the liquid portion of blood in a test tube. The aPTT is used not only to detect clotting factor deficiencies, but also used to monitor heparin's effectiveness.

ecule than LMWH. Heparin blocks both thrombin and factor Xa, whereas LMWH has relatively more activity against factor Xa and relatively less activity against thrombin. By contrast, fondaparinux acts exclusively against factor Xa—it does not affect thrombin. Fondaparinux does not require monitoring.

23. What is the initial treatment of PE?

Most patients with PE are initially admitted to the hospital. Depending on how much blood flow through the lung is blocked, symptoms of PE may be mild or severe. Besides anticoagulants, patients may require oxygen and intravenous fluids. In severe cases, patients may require not only oxygen and intravenous fluids, but also admission to an intensive care unit and treatment with powerful clot-busting drugs known as thrombolytics that actually lyse (dissolve) clots. (See Question 29.)

While LMWH is sometimes used for the initial treatment of PE, it has not been as well studied as standard heparin in this situation. Consequently, standard heparin is often the first treatment, although LMWH is being used with increasing frequency in such cases. A disadvantage of standard heparin is that it is usually administered continuously in an intravenous infusion. An advantage of this route of administration, however, is that the intravenous infusion can be turned off, allowing the heparin to disappear from the body in a few hours. This issue may be important in situations where invasive procedures (procedures that could result in bleeding, such as surgery or treatment with thrombolytic drugs) may be necessary.

When patients appear to be stable, they are usually switched from standard heparin to LMWH. This change in medications allows patients to leave the hospital sooner because they can take the LMWH at home until an oral blood thinner [warfarin (**Coumadin®**)] has taken effect.

Coumadin®

Brand name for warfarin.

24. What are the side effects of standard heparin or LMWH?

The most obvious side effect of any anticoagulant is bleeding. Bruises result from bleeding under the skin, so bruises will occur more frequently during treatment with anticoagulants. Bleeding may occur anywhere else in the body as well. Individuals may experience nosebleeds, blood in the urine, or blood in the stool. Sometimes the bleeding may be trivial. At other times, however, it may be life-threatening, especially if it occurs in the brain. The possibility of life-threatening bleeding explains why levels of anticoagulants must be monitored very closely.

The most obvious side effect of any anticoagulant is bleeding. The possibility of life-threatening bleeding explains why levels of anticoagulants must be monitored very closely.

Another side effect of either standard heparin or LMWH therapy is thinning of the bones. This complication is rarely a problem unless these medications are used at full doses for months at a time, such as is required during pregnancy.

A rare, but potentially life- (or extremity-) threatening complication of heparin is heparin-induced **thrombocytopenia**. This problem is more likely to occur with standard heparin than with LMWH. Heparin-induced thrombocytopenia results from the formation of **antibodies** against complexes of heparin and platelets. Antibodies are proteins that the body produces to attack foreign invaders, such as infections. Unfortunately, in this case the antibodies mistake the complexes of heparin and platelets for foreign cells. In the process, the antibodies activate the platelets (See Question 3) and, paradoxically, the activated platelets cause blood clots. One of the first signs of this complication is a falling number of platelets. When heparin-induced thrombocytopenia develops, it usually occurs within 15 days of starting or restarting treatment. The potential for this complication is why a platelet count is checked periodically during the first two to three weeks of treatment with heparin.

Thrombocytopenia
A low platelet count.

Antibody
A protein produced by the immune system in the body that travels in the blood and helps the body fight infection.

Other potential side effects of these medications include skin reactions. These reactions may not be due to the heparin or LMWH itself, but rather result from the benzyl alcohol that is used as a preservative in multidose vials (but not individual syringes).

25. What is warfarin?

Warfarin (Coumadin®) is an anticoagulant that can be taken by mouth. It has been used extensively for more than 50 years to prevent blood clots.

In the early 1930s, Dr. Karl Paul Link, at the University of Wisconsin, identified a component of spoiled sweet clover, dicumarol, that caused a bleeding disease in cattle. In 1939, Link, looking for a better rat poison, synthesized dicumarol and assigned the patents to the Wisconsin Alumni Research Foundation—hence the name "warfarin," a name derived from the organization's initials. Warfarin was introduced as a rat poison in 1948 and licensed in 1952.

Warfarin was thought to be unsafe for humans until a U.S. sailor tried to poison himself with this agent in 1955. After this unsuccessful suicide attempt, doctors began to think about using warfarin to treat people. One of the first patients to receive this drug as an anticoagulant was President Dwight Eisenhower, who was treated with warfarin after he suffered a heart attack in 1955. Joseph Stalin, who died with bleeding complications in 1953, may have been poisoned with warfarin, as suggested in the book *Stalin's Last Crime: The Plot Against the Jewish Doctors, 1948–1953*.

Since its adoption as medication for humans, warfarin has been widely used to treat and prevent clots. Besides the treatment and prevention of DVT and PE, it is used to prevent recurrent heart attacks and strokes and to prevent clots from forming in individuals with mechanical heart valves or the heart condition known as atrial fibrillation. With more than 20 million prescriptions being written for this drug each year, warfarin is the twentieth most commonly prescribed drug in

WARFARIN AND RAT POISON

Although warfarin was used as a rodenticide for many years, it is no longer used in rat poison. Most rats are now resistant to warfarin, so it isn't very effective at killing them. Brodifacoum, which is currently used in some rat poisons, is a drug that affects blood clotting in a way similar to warfarin. This compound has an extremely long half-life in the bloodstream, lasting up to several months. It isn't very useful as a "blood thinner" in people, however, because it tends to cause excessive anticoagulation and bleeding symptoms. Warfarin and rat poison are *not* the same thing!

Vitamin K

A vitamin that is essential to the production of the active forms of clotting factors II, VII, IX, and X in the liver.

the United States. At any given time, as much as 1 percent of the U.S. population may be taking warfarin.

26. How does warfarin work?

Warfarin, like heparin, blocks the action of various clotting factors, but it does not work in the same way that heparin does. Instead, warfarin blocks the action of **vitamin K**. Vitamin K is essential to the production of the active forms of clotting factors II, VII, IX, and X in the liver. During the formation of a clot, factor X combines with factor V to convert prothrombin (factor II) to thrombin, the clotting factor that converts fibrinogen to fibrin. (See Question 3 and Figure 1.) Through its action against vitamin K, warfarin prevents the production of normal amounts of factor X and prothrombin. It also interferes with the formation of the active form of two natural anticoagulants, protein C and protein S, although warfarin's action against clotting factors II, VII, IX, and X tends to overpower this effect. An advantage of warfarin over other anticoagulants is that it is taken orally (by mouth).

An advantage of warfarin over other anticoagulants is that it is taken orally (by mouth). Warfarin takes two to seven days to take effect, however, so it cannot be used for the initial treatment of DVT or PE.

27. Why is warfarin not used for initial treatment of DVT or PE?

Warfarin takes two to seven days to take effect and, therefore, cannot be used for the initial treatment of DVT or PE. Warfarin can, however, be started soon after heparin has been started. Heparin can be discontinued after warfarin has taken effect and its level has been measured and found to be in the therapeutic range.

Jennifer's story:

Immediately upon learning that I had a blood clot in a vein in my brain, I was admitted to a hospital that had a very reputable neurology department. The doctor informed me that a blood thinner would be used to treat the clot. I was given pain medication for my headaches, and I started to take heparin, which was given to me intravenously.

It was still a long road until everything was normal again. There was swelling on the nerve behind my right eye due to the clot, so I developed double vision. I had to take medication for that. Eventually the double vision subsided and my eyesight returned to normal. Each day was harder to face while I was still sick. I had to take antiseizure medication, which made me extremely tired.

Even though the doctors finally found the clot and were beginning to treat it, I had a very hard time with all of this, both emotionally and mentally. It was very traumatic for me to go through all of this because I was only 27 years old and I had just given birth to our daughter. All I wanted to do was to be at home with my family and have everything be normal. It was very hard to understand why all this was happening—women give birth successfully every day and it is such a common thing, but my situation was different. It was supposed to be the best of times, but it was also the worst of times.

After about two weeks in the hospital, I was able to go home. I came off the heparin and went home with Coumadin®, the pill form of blood thinner. It was such a relief to be able to finally go home and for us to enjoy our beautiful daughter. I prayed everything would be fine. My headaches had mostly subsided and the blood thinner was at the therapeutic level, where the doctors wanted it to be. I continued to have my blood drawn to check the level and saw a hematologist every few months. Seven months after I was first diagnosed, I was told the clot had dissolved. It was wonderful news. A couple of months after that, I was weaned off the seizure medication, but the hematologist told me I would need to stay on Coumadin®, because he didn't know if I would develop another clot if I came off it. So I continued to take Coumadin® for almost nine years.

28. What is a vena caval filter?

A **vena caval filter** is a filter that is placed in the inferior vena cava, the large vein that carries blood from the legs and abdomen to the heart (See Question 2). This filter acts like a sieve, allowing blood to pass but blocking clots from traveling to the lungs.

Venal caval filters are placed primarily in two situations. First, they are placed in patients with DVT or PE who have active bleeding or a very high perceived risk of bleeding, so that anticoagulation would be especially unsafe for those individuals. Second, they are placed in individuals who have recurrent DVT or PE despite adequate anticoagulation. In a few other settings, such as certain severe trauma cases in which DVT or PE has not been diagnosed but the patient is at very high risk for DVT, some physicians believe that filters should be placed preventively. Such care is individualized, however; filters are not routinely recommended except in the first two situations.

A venal caval filter is inserted in the inferior vena cava by a radiologist who has received special training. The filter is collapsed, threaded through the large veins of the neck or groin, guided into place under x-ray, and opened when it is situated in the inferior vena cava.

Vena caval filter

A device inserted to prevent PE in patients with DVT and/or PE when anticoagulants fail or cannot be used.

Venal caval filters are sometimes a temporary measure, but often they are left in place permanently. When left in place, they do not need to be checked for the presence of clots unless problems arise. Even so, anticoagulants are usually still required in conjunction with the filters.

29. What if the DVT or PE is limb- or life-threatening?

Anticoagulants do not actually lyse (dissolve) a clot. Instead, they prevent a clot from growing, which, in most cases, allows the body's own natural processes to destroy the clot over time. Sometimes, however, a DVT is so massive that the survival of the affected limb is threatened, or a PE is so massive that the individual's life is threatened. In these cases, more aggressive treatment is required. This treatment may involve a mechanical device that breaks up clots, use of powerful clot-busting drugs (thrombolytic drugs), or both. A fresh clot, which is softer than an old clot, responds the best to these treatments.

Thrombolytic drugs are given by intravenous infusion or, using a thin tube or catheter, injected directly into the clot itself. A recently developed device breaks up clots while simultaneously injecting a thrombolytic drug into the clot. The most commonly used thrombolytic drug, altepase [tissue plasminogen activator (TPA)], is a synthetic version of naturally occurring TPA, a clot-busting protein. While thrombolytics are usually effective, there is a 1 to 3 percent risk of bleeding into the brain with these drugs, which can result in a stroke or death. There is an even higher risk of other types of internal bleeding. While aggressive treatment may prevent post-phlebitic or post-thrombotic syndrome, the risk of bleeding complications limits such aggressive treatment to cases where a person's life or limb is threatened.

PART FOUR

Long-Term Treatment with Warfarin

How long will I require treatment with warfarin?

How long can warfarin be taken?

What are the risks of treatment with wafarin?

More . . .

30. How long will I require treatment with warfarin?

The optimal duration of treatment depends on the nature of the DVT or PE, whether it was a first clot, and what the person's other risk factors for recurrence are. Initial treatment is usually for a minimum of three to six months.

31. How long can warfarin be taken?

Warfarin can be taken indefinitely. The main risk of taking warfarin over a long period is the risk of bleeding.

32. What are the risks of treatment with warfarin?

Every year, 1 to 2 percent of people who take warfarin experience an episode of bleeding that is serious or life-threatening and requires transfusion or hospitalization. Half of these major bleeding episodes involve intestinal hemorrhage. In approximately 0.5 percent of people who take warfarin, bleeding occurs in the brain (intracranial hemorrhage). Bleeding in the brain can cause brain damage or death. The risk of bleeding is related to the level of anticoagulation: the higher the level of anticoagulation, the greater the risk of bleeding. The risk of clotting is also related to the level of anticoagulation: the lower the level of anticoagulation, the greater the risk of clotting. A dose of warfarin is chosen and adjusted to minimize the risks of both bleeding and clotting.

Prothrombin time (PT)

A measure of how long it takes blood to clot in a test tube. This blood test is very sensitive to the effects of warfarin, vitamin K deficiency, or liver disease.

33. Why are frequent blood tests required?

It is difficult to predict how much warfarin an individual will require to achieve an adequate level of anticoagulation. Even the same person can require a different dose at different times. The difference between an adequate dose and a dose that is too low, allowing clots to occur, or a dose that is too high, allowing bleeding to occur, is very small. Therefore, monitoring—in the form of a **prothrombin time (PT)** test—is required to check warfarin's effectiveness. Monitoring is carried out frequently, sometimes more than once a week, until a stable dose of warfarin is achieved. Monitoring may then be carried out on a monthly basis.

34. What is the prothrombin time test?

The prothrombin time (PT) test is a blood test that measures the length of time (in seconds) that it takes for clotting to occur when tissue factor and other substances are added to the liquid portion of blood (**plasma**) in a test tube (See Question 3). A normal result requires normal levels of clotting factor VII as well as factors V and X, prothrombin, and fibrinogen. In the body, when a blood vessel is injured, the exposed subendothelium allows tissue factor to be exposed to a variety of substances. Tissue factor then combines with factor VII to set off a chain reaction called the coagulation cascade. The next step in this chain reaction is the activation of factor X. Factor X and factor V work together to convert prothrombin (factor II) to thrombin, the clotting factor that converts fibrinogen to fibrin. (See Question 18.)

The PT test is used not only to detect clotting factor deficiencies, but also to monitor warfarin level. The outcome of the test is put into a standardized form by dividing the result of an individual's PT by the result of a normal control's PT. The resulting ratio is adjusted with a value calculated to correct for differences in the test reagents (the chemicals used to start the reaction), and the final ratio is called the **international normalized ratio (INR)**. The desired INR to ensure that warfarin is effective or in the therapeutic range for patients with DVT or PE is usually between 2 and 3.

35. Where do I go to have my PT or INR measured?

Usually a family doctor, internist, or other primary care provider will draw your blood and send it to a laboratory for

Plasma

The liquid part of the blood, which contains all the proteins necessary to form a blood clot, antibodies, and a variety of other components.

International normalized ratio (INR)

A measurement of the blood's ability to clot based on the prothrombin time. In a normal individual, the INR should be 1. In a patient taking warfarin therapy, the blood takes longer to form a clot in a test tube, and the INR will be higher. The desired INR for many individuals taking warfarin is in the range of 2 to 3, but some individuals with antiphospholipid syndrome are maintained at a higher INR.

analysis. Sometimes, you may be referred to a specialized anticoagulation clinic where monitoring is performed on site. At other times, especially in more complex cases, a **hematologist** will be involved, making recommendations and performing the necessary monitoring. When individuals live a long distance from a hematologist or specialized anticoagulation clinic, they may have their blood analyzed at a local hospital or laboratory and have the results faxed to their healthcare provider.

Hematologist

A physician who specializes in the study of blood disorders, such as bleeding and clotting problems, anemia, thrombocytopenia (a low number of platelets), and white blood cell disorders.

36. Can I monitor my own INR at home?

Yes, home monitors for INR testing—known as **coagulometers**—are available. At least three are currently marketed in the United States: Hemosense INRatio®, Roche Coaguchek®, and International Technidyne Corporation's ProTime® Microcoagulation System. The machines cost between $1,000 and $2,500. They require a fingerstick blood sample, and each sample requires a new test strip or cuvette (little cup). The test strips for the INRatio® and the Coaguchek® cost $3.50 to $5 apiece, and the cuvettes for the ProTime® Microcoagulation System cost $6.50 to $12.50 apiece.

Coagulometer

A device used to measure the INR for warfarin monitoring. Devices that can be used at home are available.

For self-testing, individuals measure their INR and ask their healthcare providers for the proper warfarin dose. For self-management, individuals measure their INR and adjust their own warfarin dose according to a protocol. Studies have shown that patients are just as likely to achieve warfarin levels in the correct range if they test and monitor themselves as they are if they are monitored by a specialized anticoagulation clinic. Medicare, Medicaid, and most insurance plans will pay for coagulometers for patients with mechanical heart valves but not for other patients.

Studies have shown that patients are just as likely to achieve warfarin levels in the correct range if they test and monitor themselves as they are if they are monitored by a specialized anticoagulation clinic.

37. What is vitamin K, and what does it do?

Vitamin K is an essential molecule that comes from natural sources. Humans do not make vitamin K for themselves, but rather obtain it from two sources: from food and from vitamin K production by intestinal bacteria. Vitamin K may play a role in bone health, but its most important role is in blood clotting. This vitamin is essential to the liver's production of the active forms of clotting factors II, VII, IX, and X.

38. Why must I pay attention to my intake of vitamin K while I am taking warfarin?

Warfarin blocks the action of vitamin K, but too much vitamin K can override the effects of warfarin and allow the liver to produce the active forms of clotting factors II, VII, IX, and X despite your use of warfarin. In this situation, the INR falls and the risk of clotting increases. With too little vitamin K, the INR rises and the risk of bleeding increases. For this reason, it is important to take the same amount of vitamin K every day.

David's story:

After two PEs, I am on Coumadin® for the rest of my life. I have found that living with Coumadin® and watching one's diet can be tricky. I have to get my INR checked periodically at the anticoagulation clinic, and I have to be diligent about my food intake. I had an enlightening experience after I decided that the 15 pounds I picked up during a vacation (due to lots of calories and inactivity) had to be removed quickly. I went on a crash diet. I starved myself for 72 hours (no food intake). My next INR check was 6.8! The staff at the anticoagulation clinic told me to eat some greens, hold my Coumadin® for two days, and come back to the clinic in three days. It took a while to get my INR back in the therapeutic range. I had to have my INR checked two times a week for at least two weeks. The lesson I learned from my experience was that many foods have vitamin K in them, even if they are not very high in vitamin K. Eliminating them completely can really raise the INR. I am lucky I didn't have a hemorrhage.

39. Which foods contain vitamin K?

Foods vary widely in their vitamin K content, which may range from nearly 0 micrograms per serving to more than 1,000 micrograms per serving. The foods that contain the most vitamin K are dark green, leafy vegetables. Foods that contain more than 100 micrograms per serving include leafy green vegetables, broccoli, Brussels sprouts, or foods made with these vegetables.

Physicians and anticoagulation clinics that prescribe warfarin will generally provide information about which foods are rich in vitamin K and the number of servings that are allowed per day. More information is available on the U.S. Department of Agriculture (USDA) Web site (www.ars.usda.gov/Services/docs.htm?docid=9673). Two helpful documents can be found there: "USDA National Nutrient Database for Standard Reference, Release 18—Vitamin K (Phylloquinone) (μg) Content of Selected Foods per Common Measure, Sorted by Nutrient Content" and "USDA National Nutrient Database for Standard Reference, Release 18—Vitamin K (Phylloquinone) (μg) Content of Selected Foods per Common Measure, Sorted Alphabetically."

40. While taking warfarin, is consumption of wine, beer, or liquor allowed?

Having three or more alcoholic drinks per day can interfere with warfarin. Some physicians or anticoagulation clinics advise against drinking any alcohol. Others recommend no more than one or two drinks per day. Individuals should check with their physician or anticoagulation clinic.

41. What about taking other medications while taking warfarin?

Warfarin interacts with many drugs, including both prescription and nonprescription (over-the-counter) drugs. You should check with your healthcare provider before starting, changing, or stopping any drug, including over-the-counter drugs. The healthcare provider may recommend that your INR be checked a few days later. Drugs that may interact with warfarin include heart medications; antibiotics; aspirin and other nonsteroidal anti-inflammatory drugs, such as ibuprofen (Motrin®, Advil®, Nuprin®) and naproxen (Aleve®, Orudis® KT); medications for cancer; medications for depression; medications for diabetes; medications for digestive problems such as cimetidine (Tagamet®) and ranitidine (Zantac®); medications for epilepsy, gout, high cholesterol, and thyroid problems; and vitamin supplements containing vitamin K.

Warfarin interacts with many drugs, including both prescription and nonprescription (over-the-counter) drugs.

42. What about dietary supplements and herbal medications while taking warfarin?

Not much is known about dietary supplements and herbal medications and their interactions with warfarin. Dietary supplements and herbal medication that may affect the INR and are, therefore, best avoided include arnica, bilberry, butcher's broom, cat's claw, dong quai, feverfew, forskolin, garlic, ginger, ginkgo biloba, horse chestnut, inositol hexophosphate, licorice, melilot (sweet clover), pau d'arco, red clover, St. John's wort, sweet woodruff, turmeric, willow bar, bromelains, coenzyme Q10, danshen, wheat grass, and any vitamin supplement containing vitamin K.

43. How can I reduce my risk of bleeding with warfarin without increasing my risk of a clot?

The key to minimizing the risks of bleeding and minimizing the risks of recurrent clots is keeping the INR in the correct (therapeutic) range—and the key to keeping the INR in the therapeutic range is consistency. The correct dose of warfarin should be taken every day. Many people find they have to use a reminder system, which may include a pill container and some sort of alarm. The same amount of vitamin K should be taken every day. The INR should be checked regularly.

The key to minimizing the risks of bleeding and minimizing the risks of recurrent clots is keeping the INR in the correct (therapeutic) range—and the key to keeping the INR in the therapeutic range is consistency.

Long-Term Treatment with Warfarin

47

44. Is there an alternative to warfarin for long-term treatment or prevention of DVT and PE?

In some countries, phenprocoumon and acenocoumarol—two closely related compounds that also block the action of vitamin K—are available. In the United States, however, no other oral medication (medication that can be taken by mouth) is available to treat or prevent DVT or PE except warfarin. Ximelagatran (Exanta®), a drug that directly inhibits thrombin, initially showed promise as an alternative to warfarin for the treatment and prevention of DVT and PE. Later studies revealed that ximelagatran was as effective as warfarin, but that it had the potential to cause liver damage. The drug was presented to the FDA but was not approved.

PART FIVE

Risk Factors

Which conditions increase the
likelihood of blood clots?

What is thrombophilia?

What is factor V Leiden?

More . . .

45. Which conditions increase the likelihood of blood clots?

Many conditions increase a person's risk of developing blood clots. Some conditions are avoidable; others are not. Some conditions are genetic; others develop over time.

Age

The risk of any type of blood clot increases with age. While the risk of a DVT or PE in a child may be as low as 1 in 1 million per year, the risk of a DVT or PE in an adult is 1 in 1,000 per year. The risk is lower in younger adults and higher in older adults. The risk doubles with each decade of life after age 40.

Weight

Being overweight or obese doubles a person's risk of developing a DVT or PE. Thus many Americans, 25 percent to 30 percent of whom are classified as obese, are at an increasing risk of developing a DVT or PE.

Immobility

Lupus

An autoimmune disorder characterized by multiple types of autoantibodies. Common clinical manifestations include arthritis, facial rashes, and fatigue. Many patients with lupus will have antiphospholipid antibodies, referred to as secondary antiphospholipid syndrome.

Slow, sluggish, or nonexistent blood flow increases the risk of a blood clot. Immobility probably contributes to the increased risk of blood clots associated with air travel, injury, surgery, or hospitalization as well as the increased risk of DVT or PE that arises after stroke or paralysis.

Infection

Serious infections can increase the levels of clotting factors in the blood and increase a person's risk of developing a DVT or PE.

Chronic Diseases

Chronic diseases that increase the risk of a blood clot include heart disease, cancer, **lupus,** rheumatoid arthritis, (possibly) diabetes, kidney disease, inflammatory bowel disease, sickle cell **anemia,** and leukemia.

Hospitalization

Twenty percent of all episodes of DVT and PE occur in the hospital. Hospitalization increases the risk of DVT or PE tenfold. Besides the patient's immobility, several other factors contribute to the higher incidence (number of cases) in hospitalized individuals. Infection and certain chronic diseases increase the risk of a blood clot, and people who are in the hospital are more likely to have one of these conditions. Both surgery and trauma increase the risk of blood clots. People in the hospital are also more likely to have been injured or have had an operation.

Anemia
A low red blood cell count. Anemia may be due to many causes, including low iron stores (called "iron-deficiency anemia") or antibody-mediated destruction of red blood cells (referred to as "autoimmune hemolytic anemia").

Intravenous Catheters

Intravenous catheters (thin tubes inserted into veins) can damage veins and predispose an individual to the formation of a blood clot. Because of the need for fluids and medications, people in the hospital are more likely to have had an intravenous catheter inserted.

Most intravenous catheters are inserted in superficial veins—those that lie just below the skin. Because superficial veins do not carry blood directly back to the heart, the consequences of a superficial vein thrombosis are not the same as those associated with DVT. (See Question 8.) Some intravenous catheters are inserted in larger veins that do carry blood directly back to the heart, however. Clots that form as a result of catheters in these veins can result in PE.

Trauma

Trauma increases the risk of DVT or PE tenfold. Trauma is inevitably accompanied by injury to blood vessels, which allows blood clots to form. Also, trauma increases the levels of clotting factors in the blood, which further increases the risk of blood clots. People who are recovering from trauma have the highest risk of developing a DVT or PE of any patients in the hospital.

Mike's story:

I was a triathlete and competed in 100-plus-mile bike races before my illness. In October 2003, I broke my right foot while on a long training run. Because the break was in three places, a cast was required on my right leg up to the knee. In December, a second cast was put on my leg due to discomfort in my calf after keeping my foot elevated.

While on a business trip a few days after getting the new cast, I developed flu like symptoms and unusual leg swelling. I returned home later that week feeling sick. My cast was very tight. My wife sent me to the orthopedic doctor. He removed my cast and sent me to get an ultrasound. Much to my surprise, the doctors determined that I had an extensive DVT in my right leg; the femoral and popliteal veins were occluded. After a CT scan, the doctors found that I had bilateral PEs (in both lungs). I was in serious trouble, and I was admitted into the hospital. You know that you are in bad shape when the hospital tells you not to move, asks where they can reach your wife, and asks if you would like for them to call a priest. Whenever a sentence ends in "call a priest," it is never good.

Surgery

Surgery increases the risk of DVT or PE 20-fold. Like trauma, surgery is accompanied by injury to blood vessels, which allows blood clots to form. Also, surgery increases the levels of clotting factors in the blood, further increasing the risk of blood clots.

Hormones

Men may actually have a higher overall risk of thrombosis than women, but women have some risks—namely, those associated with pregnancy, some methods of birth control, and postmenopausal hormone therapy—that men do not. Hormones, and especially **estrogen,** increase the risk of DVT and PE three- to fivefold. Estrogen is a key ingredient in birth control pills, patches, and rings, and in postmenopausal hormone therapy. Estrogen levels also increase dramatically during pregnancy.

Air Travel

Air travel increases the risk of thrombosis. Studies have shown that the risk of having DVT and PE increases dramatically after flights that last for six hours or longer. Besides immobility, other factors may explain this phenomenon. One study examined blood samples taken from the same individuals after they sat in a movie theater for eight hours compared to after they took an eight-hour plane flight. In a few individuals, measurements of clotting factor activation were higher after the eight-hour plane flight than they were after the eight hours of movies. The researchers concluded that activation of clotting factors contributes to some cases of air travel-related thrombosis.

Varicose Veins

Varicose veins contain damaged valves; as a consequence, they appear enlarged and prominent. Perhaps because of the slow or sluggish blood flow within them, varicose veins may predispose a person to the formation of blood clots. (Varicose veins can be removed or obliterated by a vascular surgeon or other specialist.)

Previous Blood Clots

The most important risk factor for having a blood clot is having had one in the past. While the overall risk for adults of having DVT or PE is 1 in 1,000 per year, the risk of having DVT or PE if one has had a blood clot in the past is 1 in 20 per year.

Estrogen

A female hormone that occurs naturally, helps sustain pregnancy, and can be synthesized. It is a key ingredient in birth control pills, patches, and rings, and in postmenopausal hormone therapy.

Studies have shown that the risk of having DVT and PE increases dramatically after flights that last for six hours or longer.

Varicose veins

Enlarged, prominent veins that result from damaged valves.

Hypercoagulable

Refers to an increased tendency to form blood clots, due to either an inherited state (for example, factor V Leiden) or an acquired disorder (for example, cancer).

Polycythemia

Too many red blood cells. If severe, polycythemia may predispose a patient to DVT.

Thrombocytosis (thrombocythemia)

Too many blood platelets. It may predispose a patient to thrombosis.

Factor V Leiden

Factor V is an important blood clotting protein. Factor V Leiden occurs when a specific mutation in the factor V gene results in a protein that is more resistant to being turned off, leading to an increased risk for forming blood clots. Factor V Leiden is the most common inherited hypercoagulable state or thrombophilia.

46. What is thrombophilia?

Thrombophilia (also known as **hypercoagulability**) is a predisposition to the development of blood clots. Thrombophilia can be either inherited or acquired during one's lifetime. Conditions leading to thrombophilia that can be acquired or develop during one's lifetime include abnormalities of the blood such as too many red blood cells (**polycythemia**) or too many platelets (**thrombocytosis** or thrombocythemia), placement of a mechanical heart valve, or the development of abnormal proteins or antibodies.

Inherited thrombophilia was first described in the 1960s, when researchers discovered the existence of antithrombin deficiency. Antithrombin is a natural anticoagulant that blocks both the conversion of prothrombin to thrombin and the conversion of factor X to its active form, factor Xa. (See Question 18.) Protein C and protein S deficiencies were described in the 1980s. Protein C and protein S are natural anticoagulants that, in combination with each other, degrade or destroy factor V. In the 1990s, **factor V Leiden** and a **mutation** in the prothrombin **gene** were also described.

Dena's story:

After I had emergency surgery for dead bowel caused by a blood clot that had formed in my superior mesenteric vein (a vein in the intestines) and was also found to have small clots that had formed in both common femoral veins (the veins in my groin), a hematologist was called in. After running some tests, he discovered that I had a rare hereditary blood disease called protein S deficiency.

I was put on lifelong Coumadin®. I have my PT and INR checked monthly at a local lab, and after being on Coumadin® for 15 years, I am at a therapeutic level and live a very normal life. I have researched this blood disease, and have since found out that several family members on my mother's side also have it. Some have been put on various blood thinners, and others are on aspirin therapy. I am so thankful that my condition was discovered in time, and that I am knowledgeable and prepared in case this disease is passed along to my daughter.

47. What is factor V Leiden?

Factor V Leiden, named after the city in the Netherlands where it was first described, is a variant of the normal clotting factor V. The gene for factor V Leiden differs from the gene for normal factor V by a single nucleotide (nucleotides are the building blocks of DNA). As a result, it produces a protein that differs by one amino acid (amino acids are the building blocks for proteins) from normal factor V. While factor V Leiden is completely normal in terms of its ability to prevent bleeding, the one amino acid difference makes factor V Leiden resistant to being degraded or inactivated by protein C and protein S. Consequently, factor V Leiden lingers in the circulation longer and, therefore, contributes to the formation of blood clots.

Individuals who have inherited one copy of the gene for factor V Leiden (heterozygotes) have a 3- to 10-fold increased risk of DVT or PE; individuals who have inherited two copies of the gene (homozygotes) have an 80- to 100-fold increased risk. Among individuals of northern European ancestry who appear to have inherited a tendency to form blood clots, 20 to 40 percent have been found to carry the factor V Leiden gene. Prior to the discovery of factor V Leiden, fewer than 10 percent of cases of thrombosis could be explained by an inherited thrombophilia.

The percentage of people who have factor V Leiden depends on the population studied. Higher percentages are reported among people of European ancestry compared to people from other continents. In the United States, factor V Leiden has been found in 5 percent of individuals of European ancestry, 2 percent of individuals of African ancestry, 2 percent of

Mutation

A change in a gene from its natural state. Mutations may cause disease or result in a normal variant that causes no problems for the patient.

Gene

The blueprints for making individual proteins, located in the DNA. The human genome codes for an estimated 20,000 to 25,000 individual genes.

Individuals who have inherited one copy of the gene for factor V Leiden (heterozygotes) have a 3- to 10-fold increased risk of DVT or PE; individuals who have inherited two copies of the gene (homozygotes) have an 80- to 100-fold increased risk.

individuals of Hispanic ancestry, 2 percent of Native Americans, and less than 1 percent of individuals of Asian ancestry.

Lori's story:

I remember the conversation as if it were yesterday. My mother shared with me the painful recollection of the loss of her son she delivered stillborn 14 months before she gave birth to me. We never talked about this sad experience again, not until 1999.

In June 1999, I was eight weeks pregnant and went to my obstetrician for my first pregnancy check-up. Before seeing the doctor, I filled out a family history form, noting that my younger brother had a blood clot in his arm, and my mother had pulmonary embolism—blood clots in the lungs. In addition, both my great aunt and her sister, who was my maternal grandmother, had blood clots in their legs. I discussed these medical findings with my doctor, and she ordered DNA testing to see if I had a genetic predisposition to clotting.

Two weeks passed, and I assumed that everything from my check-up was fine. I was wrong. My doctor called and said my DNA lab results showed that I am homozygous for a blood clotting condition called factor V Leiden. Having this disorder along with being pregnant put me at "high risk." Without medication, I could develop clots, possibly resulting in a miscarriage or stillbirth. I immediately met with a hematologist and perinatalogist to discuss my disorder.

I learned that being homozygous, which means I inherited a defective gene from both my parents, puts me at an 80 to 100 times increased risk of having a blood clot. Since my doctors did not have a lot of experience with pregnant homozygous factor V Leiden patients, my case was presented during rounds at a local hospital for review and discussion. My medical management would include daily injections of low-molecular-weight heparin during my pregnancy and post delivery.

Initially, I was scared. I was concerned the heparin would harm the baby and me. There seemed to be a general lack of information about this disorder, and I felt isolated. My fear was further exacerbated when my mother developed pulmonary embolism during my pregnancy. Fortunately, she recovered and is now managed with Coumadin® therapy.

To learn more about factor V Leiden, I read my doctor's notes, my lab tests, and articles on the Internet. I had faith in my doctors and my pregnancy went well. On January 17, 2000, my husband and I were blessed with the birth of our daughter.

Since discovering my disorder, I am enjoying life, and I try to make smart choices every day to decrease my risk of clotting. For example, I stay hydrated, I exercise, I am not on birth control pills, and I don't smoke. In addition, [this experience] has allowed me to educate my extended family regarding its effects. My mother, father, brother, daughter, aunt, and cousins were tested and have factor V Leiden. Thanks to my experience, I feel empowered to educate people, particularly women, about thrombosis and thrombophilia. In August 2003, I co-founded the National Alliance for Thrombosis and Thrombophilia (NATT).

NATT is a nationwide, community-based, voluntary health organization dedicated to preventing blood clots and ensuring that all persons suffering from blood clots and/or blood clotting disorders receive early diagnosis, optimal treatment, and quality support. NATT sustains its mission through research, education, support, and advocacy on behalf of those at risk of, or affected by, blood clots and blood clotting disorders. NATT'S Web site is www.nattinfo.org

Not only has NATT grown, but my daughter is now 6½ years old. She understands that she has a blood clotting disorder, which she calls "sticky blood." My mother is still on Coumadin® and doing well, and my cousin took heparin during her pregnancies and now has two healthy little boys. I am currently six months pregnant and taking low-molecular-weight heparin again. I have a great team of physicians. A perinatalogist and a hematologist manage my case together to ensure I am in good health.

Overall, I am very grateful my genetic disorder was identified. The death of my grandmother from a stroke, most likely the result of a clot, and the future of my family spur me on to increase awareness, research, and treatment of blood clots and blood clotting disorders. My grandmother may have had an undiagnosed clotting disorder. She died approximately 20 years before a genetic test was available. Knowledge is power. It can save lives. If nothing else, I want my children to accept having a blood clotting disorder, not to fear it.

Lori Preston, MBA
Vice President and co-founder of NATT

48. What is the prothrombin gene mutation?

Prothrombin gene G20210A mutation

An abnormality of the gene for the clotting factor, prothrombin, located at position 20210, that results in the production of more prothrombin. In individuals with this prothrombin gene mutation, prothrombin levels are higher, contributing to increased formation of blood clots.

The **prothrombin gene G20210A mutation** differs from the gene for normal prothrombin or factor II by a single nucleotide (nucleotides are the building blocks of DNA). This mutation causes the body to produce excess amounts of prothrombin. Consequently, in individuals with the prothrombin gene mutation, prothrombin levels are higher, which in turn contributes to the formation of blood clots.

Individuals who have inherited one copy of the gene (heterozygotes) have a risk of DVT or PE similar to the risk of individuals who have inherited one copy of the factor V Leiden gene.

Individuals who have inherited two copies of the prothrombin gene mutation (homozygotes) or individuals who have inherited one copy of the prothrombin gene mutation and one copy of the factor V Leiden (compound heterozygotes) have a risk of DVT or PE similar to the risk of individuals who have inherited two copies of the factor V Leiden gene.

The percentage of people who have the prothrombin gene depends on the population studied. As with factor V Leiden, higher percentages are reported among people of European descent compared to people from other continents. In the United States, the prothrombin gene mutation has been found in 1 to 2 percent of Americans of European ancestry and fewer Americans of other ancestry.

Mike's story:

After my DVT and bilateral PEs, I was put on a regimen of heparin and Coumadin® and went through three lysis procedures (with clot-busting or thrombolytic drugs) for the DVT by the interventional radiologist. Each time the procedures went extremely well, and the popliteal and common femoral veins were cleared of the clots. Even though I stayed on heparin and Coumadin, the clots came back. The results of the lysis procedures were very disappointing, and I will be on Coumadin for the rest of my life.

Later, it was determined that I had a genetic blood disorder. I am heterozygous for the prothrombin gene mutation, which I inherited from my father's side of the family.

49. What is antiphospholipid antibody syndrome?

Antiphospholipid antibody syndrome is a condition in which the body produces antibodies that target phospholipids (**antiphospholipid antibodies**). **Phospholipids** are the molecules that form the membranes of cells, including the cells that make up the endothelium, the smooth slippery surface that lines blood vessels. Antibodies are proteins produced by the body as part of its defense mechanism against foreign invaders such as infections. In the case of antiphospholipid syndrome, the antibodies attack phospholipids and damage the endothelium. (See Question 3.)

Individuals who produce such antibodies are at a high risk of developing blood clots in both arteries and veins. Pregnant women who have these antibodies are not only at increased risk of forming blood clots, but—because these antibodies may

---

Antiphospholipid antibody syndrome (APS)

A rare autoimmune disorder characterized by recurrent blood clots and/or miscarriages. By definition, people with APS have elevated antiphospholipid antibody levels in their blood. APS may occur in individuals with lupus or related autoimmune diseases, or as a primary syndrome in otherwise healthy individuals (referred to as "primary APS").

Antiphospholipid antibody

A type of autoantibody associated with an increased risk for forming blood clots (deep vein thrombosis, pulmonary embolism, stroke, and heart attack) or recurrent miscarriages. These autoantibodies generally do not bind directly to phospholipids, but instead bind to certain proteins that in turn bind to phospholipids.

59

Phospholipid

A type of fat molecule found in many locations throughout the body, including in the membranes that surround all of our cells.

Lupus anticoagulant

A type of antiphospholipid antibody that is detected through blood clotting tests, especially the activated partial thromboplastin time (aPTT). This autoantibody is associated with an increased risk for blood clots.

attack the endothelium of the blood vessels that supply the circulation to the uterus, placenta, and unborn baby—are at increased risk of miscarriage and other pregnancy complications. Other potential pregnancy complications include babies with poor growth (fetal growth restriction), premature separation of the placenta from the uterus (placental abruption), preeclampsia (high blood pressure of pregnancy), and stillbirth.

Several types of phospholipids exist, and different antibodies may be formed against the various types of phospholipids as part of antiphospholipid syndrome. Three antibodies have been shown to be associated with blood clots, miscarriage, and other pregnancy complications: anticardiolipin antibodies, anti-beta$_2$ glycoprotein I antibodies, and the **lupus anticoagulant**. The lupus anticoagulant is actually misnamed. First, most patients with lupus anticoagulants do not actually have lupus. This antibody was first described in a patient with lupus, which explains that part of the name. Second, the lupus anticoagulant is not an anticoagulant at all. As is true of anticardiolipin antibodies and anti-beta$_2$ glycoprotein I antibodies, individuals who have the lupus anticoagulant are actually at an increased risk of forming blood clots.

The term "lupus anticoagulant" comes from the behavior of plasma taken from individuals with these antibodies during a partial thromboplastin time (aPTT) test. (See Question 21.) The aPTT measures the length of time (in seconds) that it takes for clotting to occur when certain substances are added to the liquid portion of blood in a test tube (plasma). One of these substances is phospholipid. The aPTT test is prolonged when there is a deficiency of certain clotting factors or when heparin is present—two conditions that carry an increased risk for bleeding. In contrast, when the aPTT is prolonged due to interference from antibodies to phospholipids, the patient actually has an increased risk for thrombosis. The lupus anticoagulant is one of the antibodies that binds to phospholipids in this way and frequently causes the aPTT to be prolonged. While the aPTT is used to detect clotting factor deficiencies and to monitor heparin levels, it can also be used to identify antiphospholipid syndrome.

Jennifer's story:

Four years after I had the blood clot in the vein in my brain, which occurred after I had preeclampsia and had given birth to our daughter, we moved from upstate New York to North Carolina. My hematologist from upstate New York referred me to a university medical center in North Carolina where there was a hematologist who specialized in blood clotting disorders. He monitored my Coumadin® and did blood tests periodically. He told me I have antibodies in my blood that can make me more susceptible to blood clots and verified that I have antiphospholipid syndrome.

50. Can children get blood clots?

Yes, children can develop clots. Even unborn babies can have clots. Like adults, they may develop clots in their arteries or veins, with two-thirds of these clots occurring in the veins (DVT or PE). The chance of developing DVT or PE, however, is much lower in children than in adults. While the risk of DVT or PE in adults is 1 in 1000 per year, the equivalent risk in children may be as low as 1 in 1 million per year. This may be an underestimate, however, because the diagnosis is rarely suspected in children.

Most cases of DVT occur in children who have an intravenous catheter (a thin tube inserted into a vein) because of a serious medical illness. Other risk factors for DVT or PE in children include infection, heart disease, surgery, trauma, cancer, lupus, rheumatoid arthritis, diabetes, kidney disease, heart disease, sickle cell anemia, leukemia, obesity, and thrombophilia—all conditions that are also risk factors in adults. In general, because children are less likely to develop DVT or PE, multiple risk factors are usually present in children who do experience these conditions. Eighty percent of children who develop DVT or PE in the absence of any other obvious risk factor will have a thrombophilia, and frequently multiple forms of thrombophilia.

Diagnosing DVT or PE in children is not necessarily the same as it is in adults. As mentioned earlier, most cases of DVT in children are related to placement of an intravenous catheter, and intravenous catheters are typically placed in an arm or neck vein. The clots that occur in these veins are hard to see with duplex ultrasound because the ultrasound can not penetrate the bones of the chest. Given that ultrasound misses more than half of cases, magnetic resonance imaging may be necessary to make a definitive diagnosis. The preferred method to diagnose a PE in children is a VQ scan. (See Question 9.)

Because few pediatricians have experience in treating children with blood clots, children with a DVT or PE are best treated in a specialized hemostasis and thrombosis center or hemophilia treatment center.

Little research has been done on the treatment of thromboses in children. Specialists in pediatric hematology who treat children with DVT or PE tend to base their therapy on data gathered from studies involving adults. Not only has little research been done in children, but no liquid form of warfarin or pediatric doses of LMWH in pre-drawn-up syringes exist. Because few pediatricians have experience in treating children with blood clots, children with a DVT or PE are best treated in a specialized hemostasis and thrombosis center or hemophilia treatment center. The good news is that children who have been treated with warfarin for long periods of time, other than having some thinning of their bones, seem to develop normally.

PART SIX

Pregnancy

Does pregnancy cause blood clots?

Why is the use of warfarin unsafe during pregnancy?

Why is the use of heparin or LMWH
considered safe during pregnancy?

More . . .

51. Does pregnancy cause blood clots?

Pregnancy does not cause blood clots, but pregnancy does increase a woman's chance of developing a blood clot by about fourfold. A woman's risk is even higher immediately after delivery: in the first six weeks after delivery, a new mother's chance of developing a blood clot is five times higher than during her pregnancy. This tendency to form blood clots post delivery likely evolved to protect women from hemorrhage at the time of miscarriage or childbirth. Nonetheless, the chance that a young, healthy woman will develop a blood clot during pregnancy is still low, about 1 to 2 in 1,000.

Eighty percent of blood clots that arise during pregnancy occur in the veins. Four of every five venous clots involves DVT, and one of every five involves PE. The other 20 percent of blood clots occur in arteries. Five of every six arterial blood clots leads to stroke, and one of every six causes a heart attack.

Women who have had a blood clot in the past have a 1 to 2 percent risk of developing a blood clot each year. This risk increases by fourfold during pregnancy, so these women's risk of developing a blood clot during pregnancy is 5 to 10 percent. Use of anticoagulants can reduce this risk to about 1 percent. Therefore, most women who have experienced a blood clot in the past, even if they are not on anticoagulants prior to pregnancy, will be prescribed anticoagulants during pregnancy and for the six weeks after delivery. While women who had a blood clot in the past do not necessarily need to avoid pregnancy, they should be conscious of the risks to themselves and their unborn babies, consult knowledgeable physicians, and plan accordingly.

52. Why is the use of warfarin unsafe during pregnancy?

Warfarin is the most commonly prescribed and most convenient anticoagulant (because it can be taken by mouth). It is not considered safe for unborn babies, however. Warfarin crosses the placenta and has been shown to cause miscarriages in as many as 50 percent of pregnancies, birth defects in as many as 30 percent of unborn babies, internal bleeding in 2 percent of unborn babies, and neurological problems in 14 percent of children whose mothers took warfarin during pregnancy. Therefore, women are advised to avoid pregnancy while they are on warfarin. If they do become pregnant while taking this drug and plan to continue the pregnancy, they should switch to LMWH as soon as they have a positive pregnancy test.

53. Why is the use of heparin or LMWH considered safe during pregnancy?

Heparin and LMWH are considered safe in pregnancy because these drugs do not cross the placenta and, therefore, do not enter the circulation of unborn babies. In fact, in women who have thrombophilia, heparin or LMWH may actually improve the outcome of pregnancy in women who have had a previous pregnancy complicated by a poor fetal growth (fetal growth restriction), premature separation of the placenta from the uterus (placental abruption), high blood pressure of pregnancy (preeclampsia), or a stillbirth. Heparin and LMWH have been used in pregnancy by thousands of women with no increased risk of birth defects or bleeding problems in their unborn babies.

54. How are blood clots treated during pregnancy?

Blood clots are treated the same way during pregnancy as they would be outside of pregnancy, except that warfarin is rarely used. Whether women are treated initially with standard "unfractionated" heparin or LMWH, they will ultimately need to receive twice-daily injections of an anticoagulant until after delivery of the baby. Women are sometimes concerned about having to give their injections into their abdomens while they are pregnant. In fact, the needle is very short and never goes below the fatty layer of tissue under the skin.

Special plans may need to be made around the time of delivery or miscarriage in a woman with a blood clotting problem. LMWH, if it is in the mother's system at the time of miscarriage or childbirth, or when an epidural or spinal anesthetic is desired, may increase the risk of bleeding complications. Therefore, standard or "unfractionated" heparin, which is shorter acting, may be used during the last few weeks of pregnancy and held at the time of delivery. Alternatively, LMWH may be continued and withheld in anticipation of delivery or surgery for miscarriage. LMWH can be resumed after delivery. One or two weeks after delivery, when the risk of major bleeding has subsided, women can be converted to warfarin for the remainder of their treatment.

55. How are blood clots prevented during pregnancy?

Blood clots are prevented with anticoagulants and other measures. Except in rare cases, warfarin is not used. Women who are taking warfarin to prevent blood clots should switch to LMWH before they become pregnant or should switch to LMWH as soon as they have a positive pregnancy test. They will need twice-daily injections of this drug until after delivery of the baby. (See Question 54.) One or two weeks after delivery, when the risk of major bleeding has subsided, women can be converted back to warfarin.

Women who were not taking warfarin prior to pregnancy, but who have had a blood clot in the past, will usually need to take LMWH during pregnancy. They will likely not need a full dose, unlike someone who was being treated for a blood clot or someone who was taking warfarin before pregnancy. In fact, sometimes these women will need only one daily injection. Because pregnancy causes LMWH to be cleared from the circulation more quickly, however, most women will still need two injections per day. The same precautions are required at the time of miscarriage or childbirth as are required for women who are taking a full dose of LMWH. Because LMWH may increase the risk of bleeding complications if it is in the mother's system at the time of miscarriage or childbirth, or when an epidural or spinal anesthetic is desired, a low dose of standard "unfractionated" heparin, which is shorter acting, may be substituted for LMWH during the last few weeks of pregnancy and held at the time of delivery. Alternatively, LMWH may be continued and withheld in anticipation of delivery or surgery for miscarriage. The LMWH can be resumed after delivery and continued for the six weeks after delivery while the risk of a blood clot is still relatively high.

Pregnant women do not need to follow a special diet as part of a plan to avoid blood clots. Instead, they should follow the advice of their obstetric providers regarding diet and avoid becoming dehydrated. Avoiding dehydration is especially important during the first three months of pregnancy, when women are most susceptible to nausea and vomiting. Extreme nausea and vomiting in early pregnancy, which is known as hyperemesis gravidarum, requires treatment with intravenous fluids. Perhaps because dehydration increases the concentration of clotting factors in the blood, women with hyperemesis gravidarum are two to three times more likely to develop DVT or PE than other pregnant women.

No special exercises are required to avoid blood clots. Again, women should follow the advice of their obstetric providers. Given that immobility and air travel are known risk factors for DVT and PE, pregnant women should move around every two hours when they are on a trip. Women who are on bed rest for vaginal bleeding or preterm labor can still move their legs and are usually encouraged to do so. This factor may explain why women who are hospitalized during pregnancy do not seem to be at an increased risk of blood clots compared to other pregnant women.

Jennifer's story:

We always wanted to have a second child, but because I had had preeclampsia and the blood clot in the vein in my brain after giving birth to our daughter, we knew I would be at risk for problems, so we didn't know if a second child would be possible. The hematologist in upstate New York told me getting pregnant would be like playing Russian roulette, and he did not recommend it.

During one of my visits with my new hematologist in North Carolina, he informed me there was a doctor at the same university medical center who dealt with high-risk pregnancies, particularly those requiring Lovenox® and heparin injections. Then we met with the high-risk obstetrician. She explained to us that women with antiphospholipid syndrome can take Lovenox® and heparin shots in the stomach throughout pregnancy and usually deliver a normal, healthy baby. The molecules in the Lovenox and heparin shots do not cross the placenta and do not cause birth defects. It is still a high-risk pregnancy and there is potential for bleeding, but it is possible to have a successful pregnancy.

We were excited and hesitant at the same time. We did finally decide to proceed. I had a very good and healthy pregnancy. There were a lot of times that I was scared, but I had faith that everything would work out well. My husband, my family, the doctors, and my friends were very supportive. It feels like it was fate to do this because we moved to North Carolina where I was treated by excellent doctors. If we had stayed in upstate New York, I think things would have been much different. Our wonderful son was born three years ago. I have learned that every day is a gift.

56. What precautions are taken at the time of delivery?

Precautions are taken to prevent hemorrhage at the time of delivery. To avoid having anticoagulation in the mother's system at the time of delivery, heparin is usually withheld (or the dose substantially reduced) 6 to 24 hours prior to the anticipated time of delivery, or as soon as labor starts.

The biggest risk of bleeding after delivery is from the uterus. After childbirth, the placenta, which is approximately 7 inches in diameter, separates from the uterus, leaving behind a large surface of open blood vessels. Hemorrhage is prevented by contractions of the uterus (which is actually a muscle). Although the primary cause of hemorrhage at the time of childbirth is failure of the uterus to contract, anticoagulation can contribute to the risk of hemorrhage. In particular, women are at an increased risk of hemorrhage if they require a cesarean delivery. Twenty-nine percent of women in the United States deliver by cesarean section. Having this procedure doubles the risk of bleeding at the time of delivery. The average woman loses a pint of blood with vaginal delivery, but two pints with a cesarean delivery. Anticoagulation can, therefore, contribute to the increased risk of bleeding with cesarean delivery.

Precautions are also taken to protect women from bleeding associated with administration of an epidural or spinal anesthetic. An epidural anesthetic provides pain relief during labor. To administer this medication, a catheter (thin tube) is placed into the epidural space, which is just outside of the dura, or wrapping, around the spinal cord; repeated or continuous doses of a local anesthetic or narcotic pain reliever are then delivered through this catheter. In contrast, a spinal anesthetic provides anesthesia for cesarean delivery. Its administration involves a single injection of a local anesthetic into the spinal fluid, which is located beneath the dura and surrounds the spinal cord.

Because bleeding in the epidural space or spinal fluid could compress the spine and cause paralysis, anesthesiologists usually refrain from giving a patient an epidural or spinal anesthetic unless a woman has been off heparin for more than 6 hours or off LMWH for more than 12 hours. If a woman needs pain relief in labor and has heparin or LMWH in her system, narcotic pain relievers are used instead of an epidural. If she requires a cesarean delivery and has heparin or

To avoid having anticoagulation in the mother's system at the time of delivery, heparin is usually withheld (or the dose substantially reduced) 6 to 24 hours prior to the anticipated time of delivery, or as soon as labor starts.

LMWH in her system, a general anesthetic is used instead of a spinal.

Precautions are taken to prevent clots while women are off anticoagulation at the time of delivery. For example, these patients may wear sequential compression devices, which wrap around the legs like blood pressure cuffs, are attached to a pump, and inflate periodically. These devices should remain in place until anticoagulation is restarted.

57. When are anticoagulants restarted after delivery?

LMWH is the preferred option following childbirth and is usually restarted 12 to 24 hours after delivery. A woman who was on a low dose during pregnancy may resume a low dose after delivery, whereas a woman who was on a full dose may resume a full dose after delivery. A woman who will require anticoagulation only for the six weeks after delivery may stay on LMWH for the entire six weeks. LMWH requires less monitoring and fewer trips to the physician's office or anticoagulation clinic than warfarin—an important consideration when a woman is trying to recover from childbirth and care for a newborn. A woman who will ultimately be resuming warfarin therapy may be converted to warfarin when the risk of bleeding has subsided, usually one to two weeks after delivery.

58. Are anticoagulants safe to take while breastfeeding?

Anticoagulants are safe to take while breastfeeding. If a mother is taking heparin or LMWH, neither appears in breast milk. If a mother is taking warfarin, a small amount may appear in breast milk, but its presence has never been shown to affect a baby. The American Academy of Pediatrics endorses breastfeeding for the babies of mothers who take warfarin.

PART SEVEN

Menstruation and Birth Control

Is it true that birth control pills cause blood clots?

Can a woman take birth control pills if she
has had a blood clot in the past?

What if a woman has thrombophilia but
has never developed a blood clot?

More . . .

59. Is it true that birth control pills cause blood clots?

Birth control pills are the leading method of birth control (contraception) in the United States. Although they do not *cause* blood clots, most birth control pills do increase a woman's chance of developing a blood clot by about three to four times.

Most oral contraceptives contain an estrogen and a progestin (synthetic progesterone). Estrogen and progesterone have many effects on a woman's body. They are the hormones that sustain pregnancy and, when given in the form of birth control pills, imitate pregnancy, thereby preventing pregnancy. These hormones also increase the levels of clotting factors and are assumed to be responsible for women's increased risk of blood clots during pregnancy.

For the average woman taking birth control pills, the absolute risk of a blood clot is very small: Only 1 in 1,000 women per year who are taking birth control pills will develop such a clot. For a woman with thrombophilia or a history of thrombosis, however, this risk is significantly higher. The new patches (transdermal contraceptives) may increase this risk even more. The amount of estrogen absorbed from the patches has been reported to be 60 percent higher than the amount delivered by the pills. Little information about the risk of blood clots with birth control rings is available. Like patches and most birth control pills, these devices also contain an estrogen and a progestin; thus they probably carry a risk of thrombosis similar to that of birth control pills or patches.

The risk of a blood clot is reduced by anticoagulation, so women who are taking anticoagulants may take birth control pills. Women who are not taking anticoagulants have limited choices for contraception, but alternative methods are available. One option is a progestin-only contraceptive. Progestin-only contraceptives include progestin-only birth

Although they do not cause blood clots, most birth control pills do increase a woman's chance of developing a blood clot by about three to four times. The hormones found in these pills—especially estrogen—are also assumed to be responsible for women's increased risk of blood clots during pregnancy.

control pills such as Micronor®, Nor-Q.D.®, and Ovrette®; the levonorgestrel (Mirena®) intrauterine device (IUD); and every-three-month injections of medroxyprogesterone acetate (Depo-Provera®). While progestin in the higher doses used to treat abnormal vaginal bleeding has been shown to increase the risk of thrombosis five- to sixfold, progestin in the doses used in contraceptives has not been shown to increase the risk of DVT or PE.

60. Can a woman take birth control pills if she has had a blood clot in the past?

The risk is of a blood clot is reduced by anticoagulation, so women who are taking anticoagulants may take birth control pills. Women who are not taking anticoagulants and have experienced a blood clot in the past are at high risk of recurrent thrombosis. For this reason, they should not use patches, rings, or birth control pills that contain estrogen. They may use progestin-only contraceptives such as Micronor®, Nor-Q.D.®, and Ovrette®; the levonorgestrel (Mirena®) intrauterine device (IUD); and every-three-month injections of medroxyprogesterone acetate (Depo-Provera®).

61. What if a woman has thrombophilia but has never developed a blood clot?

Women with thrombophilia are at increased risk of developing blood clots; in fact, the risk of a thrombosis in women with thrombophilia exceeds 1 in 100 per year. Use of birth control pills containing an estrogen and a progestin increases a woman's chance of developing a blood clot by another three to four times. For this reason, most women with thrombophilia should not use a birth control method that contains estrogen. They may use progestin-only contraceptives such as Micronor®, Nor-Q.D.®, and Ovrette®; the levonorgestrel (Mirena®) intrauterine device (IUD); and every-three-month injections of medroxyprogesterone acetate (Depo-Provera®).

62. Can anticoagulation cause heavy periods or other gynecological problems?

Women who take anticoagulants are vulnerable to heavy menstrual bleeding and bleeding into the ovary or into the abdomen at the time of ovulation (mid-cycle release of an egg). Half of women who take anticoagulants experience heavy menstrual bleeding. A smaller percentage experience bleeding into the ovary. Heavy menstrual bleeding is not a reason to discontinue anticoagulants, however, as it can be managed effectively. (See Question 63.)

Bleeding into the ovary is an infrequently considered complication of anticoagulant therapy. Ovulation is not normally accompanied by any significant amount of bleeding, but in a woman on anticoagulants, the potential exists for bleeding into the abdomen. Hormonal contraceptives that contain an estrogen/progestin combination (pills, patches, and rings) prevent ovulation and effectively prevent bleeding into the ovary. This is one reason why women who are taking anticoagulants should be allowed to take birth control pills.

63. How can heavy menstrual bleeding be managed?

If a woman is on anticoagulation, the full range of treatments to manage heavy periods may be tried. The woman will first be evaluated by a gynecologist to make sure there is no abnormality of the uterus or its lining. If an abnormality is detected, surgery may be required to correct it. If there is no abnormality, hormonal treatments may be tried. Given that birth control pills and the Mirena® intrauterine device (IUD) reduce heavy periods, one or the other may be prescribed. If a woman does not plan to have any more children, she may have the lining of her uterus destroyed by a technique called endometrial ablation or even undergo a hysterectomy. Because anticoagulation should be discontinued at the time of an operation, special planning is required if any surgery is performed. (See Question 72.)

If a woman is not on anticoagulation, her choice of treatments is more limited. The first step is still an evaluation by a gynecologist to make sure there is no abnormality of the uterus or its lining. If an abnormality is detected, surgery may be required to correct it. If there is no abnormality, hormonal treatments are limited to progestins in contraceptive doses such as Micronor®, Nor-Q.D.®, and Ovrette®; the levonorgestrel (Mirena®) IUD; and every-three-month injections of medroxyprogesterone acetate (Depo-Provera®). If a woman does not plan to have any more children, she may have an endometrial ablation or hysterectomy. Because any operation increases the risk of a blood clot, planning is required if any surgery is performed. (See Question 72.)

PART EIGHT

Menopause and Hormone Therapy

Does estrogen cause blood clots?

Can a woman who has had a blood clot
in the past take estrogen?

More . . .

64. Does estrogen cause blood clots?

Estrogen is used to treat postmenopausal symptoms such as hot flashes and vaginal dryness. Although it does not cause blood clots, estrogen does increase a woman's chance of developing a blood clot by two- to fourfold. Most postmenopausal hormone therapies contain both an estrogen and a progestin (synthetic progesterone). Estrogen and progesterone have many effects on a woman's body, including increasing the levels of clotting factors. For the average woman taking postmenopausal hormone therapy, the absolute risk of a blood clot is small: Only one in 300 women per year who are taking postmenopausal hormone therapy will develop a blood clot. This risk is much higher for a woman who has had a previous blood clot or a woman with thrombophilia.

Postmenopausal hormone therapy with estrogen, or with a combination of estrogen and a progestin, appears to increase a woman's risk of developing breast cancer, stroke, DVT, and PE.

65. Can a woman who has had a blood clot in the past take estrogen?

Studies have shown that postmenopausal hormone therapy with estrogen, or with a combination of estrogen and a progestin, increases the risk of breast cancer, stroke, DVT, and PE. For this reason, postmenopausal hormone therapy should be taken only when absolutely necessary, primarily for severe symptoms. For women who are not taking anticoagulants and have developed a blood clot in the past, as well as for women who are at an increased risk of having blood clots due to thrombophilia, the circumstances that would justify taking postmenopausal hormone therapy are rare or nonexistent.

PART NINE

Medical Problems

What if cancer is present?

What if kidney failure is present?

What if heart disease is present?

More . . .

66. What if cancer is present?

Patients with cancer are at increased risk of developing blood clots. The risk of developing blood clots varies with the type of cancer and is highest with cancers affecting the brain, pancreas, and lungs. Patients with cancer who develop blood clots also have an increased risk for other adverse outcomes—including death—compared to patients with cancer who do not have blood clots.

Other variables may also increase the risk for blood clots in patients with cancer. For example, many of these patients undergo surgery as part of their cancer treatment plan. Patients who undergo surgery have an increased risk for blood clots in general, and this risk rises even more if the patient also has cancer. Many patients receiving chemotherapy treatments for cancer will have intravenous catheters placed in one of the large veins in the neck (jugular) or under the collarbone (subclavicular), and these catheters may contribute to formation of a clot. Lastly, some chemotherapy treatments are associated with a higher risk of blood clots, including thalidomide, which is used to treat multiple myeloma, and avastin, which is used to treat colon cancer.

Patients with cancer need to receive treatment to prevent thrombosis whenever they are in the hospital, but no evidence indicates that these same treatments can prevent clots in patients who are not hospitalized. Also, although some earlier studies suggested that a low-dose regimen of warfarin might help keep catheter lines open in patients with cancer, this practice is currently not recommended by the American College of Chest Physicians (an organization that periodically publishes comprehensive guidelines on the prevention, diagnosis, and treatment of DVT and PE).

Most patients who develop a blood clot are treated with intravenous or subcutaneous therapy (heparin or LMWH) for about a week, even as they are being started on an oral medication (warfarin) for long-term treatment. (See Part 3,

Initial Treatment—Questions 15–29.) Recent studies show that patients with cancer do better if they are treated with LMWH instead of warfarin for at least the first three months of treatment. Some studies suggest that LMWH might actually contribute to an improved outcome from the cancer, but additional research is needed to confirm these results. For patients with an intravenous line in a large (central) vein who develop a clot around the catheter, the catheter should be removed if at all possible.

After a standard course of therapy with anticoagulants (the usual length of treatment is 3 to 6 months, or up to 12 months in certain circumstances), patients with cancer are at high risk for recurrent blood clots. Consequently, it is generally recommended that patients with cancer who have experienced a previous DVT or PE should continue to take an anticoagulant as long as the cancer is present or as long as they continue to receive treatment for the cancer.

Vena caval filters have also been used in patients with thrombosis and cancer who are at a high risk for bleeding and cannot safely use anticoagulants to prevent PE. (See Question 28.) Because these filters can lead to an increased risk of blood clots, these patients should continue to take anticoagulants if possible.

It is generally recommended that patients with cancer who have experienced a previous DVT or PE should continue to take an anticoagulant as long as the cancer is present or as long as they continue to receive treatment for the cancer.

67. What if kidney failure is present?

People with kidney failure have a tendency to bleed, probably because their platelets do not work as well as the platelets in people without such disease. People with kidney failure may also develop blood clots—but their tendency to bleed can make use of anticoagulants problematic. (In the discussion here, *kidney failure* refers to the need for dialysis; *kidney insufficiency* refers to abnormal kidney function, but not to the point that dialysis is required.)

A common complication encountered in people with kidney failure who are being treated with hemodialysis (filtering of the blood) is thrombosis of the catheter, graft, or fistula that is used to access the blood. For people with catheters, an anticoagulant such as heparin is generally used to keep the catheter from closing due to clotting between dialysis sessions. If such a problem does arise, clot-busting drugs that can actually dissolve the clot, such as tissue plasminogen activator (TPA), may be administered. TPA converts **plasminogen** to plasmin, which is the blood protein responsible for cutting fibrin and helping to dissolve blood clots (See Question 9). If a graft or fistula is closed by a clot, it can sometimes be reopened by using a catheter, although that approach does not always work.

People with kidney failure may also develop blood clots that are not associated with their hemodialysis access sites. The diagnosis and treatment of blood clots in these patients are similar to the approaches used in patients with normal kidney function, with a few exceptions.

First, for patients with kidney insufficiency, the contrast dye used with CT scans, arteriograms, and venography may sometimes cause problems. (See Questions 9 and 14.) In these patients, the contrast dye may worsen kidney function dramatically, eventually leading to complete kidney failure. If these patients should develop symptoms of DVT or PE, tests that do not require contrast dye should be used to diagnose the problem. For example, if DVT is suspected, an ultrasound should be performed; if PE is suspected, a VQ scan should be used rather than a spiral CT. If it is necessary and available, MRI is a safe alternative as well.

Second, some of the medicines used for the initial treatment of a blood clot are cleared by the kidney, including the LMWH preparations (enoxaparin, dalteparin, and tinzaparin). In people with kidney insufficiency, these medicines should be administered with caution and the dose decreased depending on the person's level of kidney function. In some cases, monitoring blood levels can help prevent excessive

Plasminogen

A substance naturally produced by the body that helps to break down blood clots. The active form of plasminogen is called plasmin.

anticoagulation. In general, people with kidney failure should not take LMWH unless they are under the direct care of a hematologist or other specialist who is well trained in the management of these medicines in people with kidney failure.

Third, taking warfarin is complicated by the need for INR monitoring. (See Question 34.) For people with kidney failure who receive dialysis through a catheter, the blood sample for the INR measurement should not be drawn through the catheter, because the heparin used to keep the catheter open might interfere with the blood test.

Lastly, as noted earlier, people with kidney failure tend to bleed, and anticoagulants can make this problem significantly worse. Problems with bleeding need to be considered whenever a person with kidney failure takes an anticoagulant.

68. What if heart disease is present?

People with heart disease may have a variety of problems that can lead to difficulties with the diagnosis and treatment of blood clots. Congestive heart failure, for example, increases the risk of DVT. In the past, heart attacks have been shown to increase the risk of DVT. Today, however, patients who experience a heart attack are aggressively treated with blood thinners, so DVT and PE are less common in these individuals now than they once were. Other forms of heart disease have not been proven to increase a person's risk for DVT or PE.

Atrial Fibrillation

Atrial fibrillation is characterized by an abnormal heart rhythm that leads to formation of clots within the heart; it is also associated with an increased risk for a stroke or embolism to an artery in an arm or a leg. This condition is also frequently treated with warfarin; once started, this therapy is continued indefinitely. Medicines to help regulate the heart rhythm (such as amiodarone) are frequently prescribed for atrial fibrillation

Atrial fibrillation
An abnormal rhythm or heartbeat pattern involving the atria or the upper chambers of the heart (as opposed to the ventricles or lower chambers of the heart). The abnormal rhythm can interrupt the normal flow of blood through the heart, allowing clots to form that can then travel through arteries, lodge in the brain, and cause strokes.

as well. These medicines require close monitoring of the INR whenever they are started or if the dose is changed.

Mechanical Heart Valves

People with mechanical heart valves require lifelong anticoagulation to prevent blood clots from forming on the valve—such clots could potentially break loose and cause a stroke or an embolism to an artery in an arm, leg, or other part of the body. The target INR for people with mechanical heart valves is in the range of 2.5 to 3.5, which is higher than the target set for people with DVT or PE. For some people with mechanical heart valves, a daily aspirin is added to the warfarin regimen, which can contribute to the risk for bleeding complications. People with bioprosthetic heart valves (pig valves) do not need anticoagulants.

Coronary Artery Disease and Heart Attacks

People with coronary artery disease (atherosclerosis of the arteries that supply the heart) may take medications on a chronic basis to decrease their chances of experiencing a heart attack. Some of these medications may interfere with warfarin, although this is rarely a particularly difficult problem. Many such patients will also undergo a procedure in which a stent (a thin tube) is inserted into a coronary artery to keep it open. These patients need to be treated with aspirin and clopidogrel (Plavix®) for an extended period of time. Taking warfarin, aspirin, and clopidogrel at the same time can be problematic, because the risk of bleeding complications is high with this combination.

Heart Failure

People with severe heart failure are at risk not only of DVT, but also of formation of blood clots within the heart that might potentially break loose and cause a stroke. Warfarin is sometimes used to prevent clots in people with heart failure. These individuals often take several other medications, which can complicate the management of their warfarin levels.

69. What if diabetes is present?

Diabetes is not generally regarded as a major risk factor for DVT and PE. Diabetes can damage blood vessels and may result in problems that decrease mobility. In most studies of DVT and PE, however, diabetes has not been shown to be a risk factor for blood clotting problems.

Diabetes is not generally regarded as a major risk factor for DVT and PE.

People with diabetes frequently have other health problems, which can complicate their treatment with anticoagulants. For example, these individuals may have kidney problems, which might limit their ability to use certain medicines (for example, LMWH) or lead to an increased risk for bleeding. (People with kidney failure have a tendency to bleed, probably because their platelets do not work as well as the platelets in people without kidney disease.) In general, people with diabetes do not seem to have more problems taking warfarin than people who do not have diabetes.

70. What if liver disease is present?

People with liver disease, such as hepatitis or cirrhosis, do not have an increased risk of DVT or PE compared to individuals without liver disease. Because the liver is responsible for the production of most clotting factors, people with severe liver disease have a tendency to bleed. In addition, people with cirrhosis of the liver will frequently have an enlarged spleen. The spleen becomes enlarged when an obstruction to blood flow in the liver occurs, causing a backup of blood into the spleen. An enlarged spleen can capture platelets, leading to a decrease in their overall number. Low platelets, in turn, can increase the person's risk for bleeding. Even though individuals with liver disease have a tendency to bleed, this does not prevent them from developing blood clots!

A significant issue for people with liver disease who develop DVT or PE is the choice of treatment. These individuals already have a tendency to bleed, and anticoagulants may exacerbate this problem. Such patients need to be monitored closely and have their platelet counts checked frequently. Because the risk of bleeding may be too high, they may require other treatments, such as placement of an inferior vena caval filter to prevent clots from traveling to their lungs. (See Question 28.)

On rare occasions, some people may develop clots in the veins to and from the liver. For example, the portal vein receives blood from the intestines and spleen; it then carries this blood to the liver. Clots in this vein can lead to an enlarged spleen, esophageal varices (dilated veins in the esophagus, which may bleed), and abdominal pain. In contrast, the hepatic veins drain blood from the liver into the inferior vena cava. Clots in these veins can cause swelling of the liver and abdominal pain, a disorder referred to as **Budd-Chiari syndrome.** Both inherited thrombophilia (factor V Leiden, for example) and acquired thrombophilia (abnormalities of the blood such as too many platelets or too many red blood cells) are associated with thrombosis of the portal or hepatic veins. The best treatment for patients with clots in the portal or hepatic veins is unclear, but some experts recommend indefinite anticoagulant therapy.

71. What if high blood pressure is present?

Hypertension (high blood pressure) may affect as many as one-fourth of all individuals in the United States. This condition is associated with an increased risk for heart attacks and strokes—both problems affecting the arteries. Several studies have shown that high blood pressure does not increase the risk of DVT and PE. Nevertheless, hypertension affects an increasing percentage of people as they age, so it is frequently encountered in people who have blood clots. Although both conditions may be present in the same person, one does not appear to cause the other.

People with hypertension may take a variety of medications to control their blood pressure. While none of these medications

Budd-Chiari syndrome

Thrombosis of the hepatic veins (veins coming from the liver), usually presenting with abdominal pain, enlargement of the liver, and ascites (fluid in the abdomen).

Hypertension

High blood pressure.

Hypertension may affect as many as one-fourth of all individuals in the United States, but does not appear to increase a person's risk of developing DVT and PE.

has been identified as having particularly bad interactions with warfarin, people who take warfarin should get their INR rechecked soon after starting any new medication or changing the dose of a medication that they are already taking. Many older patients with hypertension also take an aspirin each day, as a means to decrease their risk for stroke or a heart attack. Taking aspirin in addition to warfarin can increase a person's risk for bleeding complications and is recommended only if it offers a clear benefit.

PART TEN

Surgery and Trauma

What happens if I am on warfarin
and I have to have surgery?

What if I am taking warfarin and I need
emergency surgery or am injured?

How will I be protected from blood clots at the time
of surgery or injury if I am not taking warfarin?

More . . .

72. What happens if I am on warfarin and I have to have surgery?

Special plans have to be made if you need surgery. Once warfarin is discontinued, it takes approximately four to five days for its effects to disappear. If warfarin is not discontinued, bleeding may occur at your incision sites. If warfarin is discontinued, there is an increased risk of DVT or PE. Individuals who are at particularly high risk of thrombosis may be admitted to the hospital for intravenous heparin during the time they are not on warfarin or may be prescribed twice-daily LMWH to take at home (sometimes referred to as "bridging therapy"). People who are not required to take heparin or LMWH in the interim will simply stop their warfarin five days before surgery. During this time, the INR is expected to fall below 1.5 and surgery is considered safe.

Some surgeries result in very little bleeding and are considered safe to have even without stopping warfarin. While not all eye surgery falls into this category, cataract surgery is considered safe without stopping warfarin. Gastrointestinal endoscopic procedures—that is, procedures that involve examining the esophagus, stomach, or intestines with long, flexible instruments that allow the examiner to see inside these organs— include upper endoscopies, colonoscopies, and sigmoidoscopies. They may be performed without stopping warfarin, even if a small biopsy (removal of a tissue sample) is required. If any kind of surgery has to be performed at the same time as one of these procedures (such as removal of a polyp), however, warfarin should be discontinued in advance. With the exception of gum surgery, most dental procedures are considered safe to have without stopping warfarin. To prevent bleeding, dentists sometimes use a mouthwash that contains a medication that prevents clots from breaking down.

Minor surgeries on the skin, such as biopsies, are also considered safe to have without stopping warfarin. Procedures that require only a needle, such as an injection or aspiration (withdrawal of fluid), are often considered safe to have without stopping warfarin. If the needle is being used for a biopsy of the liver or a tumor or to drain fluid from deep within the abdomen, however, the patient must stop the warfarin prior to the procedure.

No matter what the surgery, both the surgeon or doctor who will be performing the procedure and the doctor or anticoagulation clinic that prescribed the warfarin should be consulted well in advance. Prior to some major operations, the INR may be checked to ensure that it is at an acceptable level. What constitutes an "acceptable" level will vary depending on the procedure being performed. After the procedure, the surgeon or doctor who performed the surgery will decide when it is safe to restart anticoagulation.

73. What if I am taking warfarin and I need emergency surgery or am injured?

In case of emergency surgery or a serious injury, the effects of warfarin must be reversed quickly. The quickest way to do so is to replace the body's clotting factors with plasma, the liquid portion of blood that contains the clotting factors. **Fresh frozen plasma,** which is kept frozen in blood banks until it is needed, is defrosted and transfused in such a case. Usually, two units are transfused and then the INR is checked to determine if more is required.

Vitamin K may also be used to reverse the effects of warfarin, but it takes 24 hours to work. Both 1 milligram of vitamin K given intravenously and half of a 5-milligram tablet taken by mouth have been shown to be effective at reducing the INR. Therefore, if surgery must be performed urgently but not within the next 24 hours, vitamin K may be used to reverse the effects of warfarin.

No matter what the surgery, both the surgeon or doctor who will be performing the procedure and the doctor or anticoagulation clinic that prescribed the warfarin should be consulted well in advance.

Fresh frozen plasma

The quickest way to reverse warfarin is to replace clotting factors. This is done with fresh frozen plasma; plasma is the liquid portion of blood that contains the clotting factors.

74. How will I be protected from blood clots at the time of surgery or injury if I am not taking warfarin?

Several strategies are used to prevent blood clots at the time of surgery or injury. The simplest strategies—and ones that do not increase the risk of bleeding—are fitted elastic compression stockings and sequential compression devices. The latter devices wrap around the legs like blood pressure cuffs, are attached to a pump, and inflate periodically. Sequential compression devices should be placed prior to surgery or at the time of injury and remain in place until anticoagulation is restarted. After surgery or injury, patients are encouraged to get out of bed as soon as it is safe to do so and asked to walk around to prevent slow or sluggish blood flow, a risk factor for the formation of blood clots.

An alternative to full anticoagulation is low doses of heparin, LMWH, or fondaparinux. Low doses of these medications do not carry the same bleeding risk as full doses. This regimen can be maintained until full anticoagulation is restarted, and it can be used for individuals who do not require full anticoagulation. Low doses of heparin, LMWH, or fondaparinux are usually started 24 hours after surgery or injury. For individuals who will be resuming warfarin therapy, full anticoagulation is restarted when the risk of serious bleeding has subsided. Warfarin may be restarted the day after surgery or postponed for some time. In the meantime, the heparin, LMWH, or fondaparinux therapy is continued at low doses or increased to full doses.

Sometimes surgery is required or an injury occurs when a person's risk of a blood clot is exceptionally high or a blood clot is already present. In these cases, a vena caval filter may be placed to prevent a PE. (See Question 28.)

PART ELEVEN

Travel

What measures can be taken to prevent
blood clots during travel?

How is anticoagulation managed during travel?

More . . .

75. *What measures can be taken to prevent blood clots during travel?*

Air travel increases the risk of thrombosis. Besides immobility, other factors may play into this increased risk (See Question 45); nevertheless, immobility is probably the single most important factor in travel-related thrombosis. Immobility—that is, lack of movement—can result in slow, sluggish, or nonexistent blood flow, which increases a person's risk of a blood clot. Therefore, the most important measure to prevent blood clots during travel is to move around for at least five minutes every two hours. Even when passengers are confined to their seats in a plane, they can still move their feet and legs. Passengers can move their feet back and forth as if stepping on and off of a gas pedal and can move their legs back and forth by bending at their knees.

Dehydration can increase the concentration of clotting factors in the blood, so staying hydrated is also important. Drinking water is recommended. (Alcohol has a dehydrating—rather than hydrating—effect.)

Fitted elastic compression stockings may also help reduce the risk of a blood clot. In one study, volunteers who were taking a flight of more than eight hours' duration were randomly assigned to one of two groups. Members of one group wore knee-high fitted elastic compression stockings; members of the other group did not. After returning from their trips, the volunteers had an ultrasound examination of their legs even though they had no symptoms of DVT. Ten percent of the group who did not wear stockings had asymptomatic DVT (DVT without any symptoms) in the calf, whereas none of the group who wore fitted elastic stockings developed DVT.

Individuals who have had DVT or PE in the past, have thrombophilia, have had recent surgery, or have other medical conditions that place them at risk such as heart failure, but who are not currently taking warfarin, should consult their physician

The most important measure to prevent blood clots during travel is to move around for at least five minutes every two hours, whether you are planning long trips by air, in the car, or on the train.

or anticoagulation clinic for recommendations prior to travel. Some physicians or anticoagulation clinics may recommend taking a single dose of a LMWH prior to flights that will last six hours or longer.

Long automobile or train trips may pose similar risks to air travel. The same precautions as for air travel should be considered when planning long trips in the car or on the train. Taking a brief, five minute walk every two hours is advised.

76. How is anticoagulation managed during travel?

Individuals who are taking warfarin should consult their physician or anticoagulation clinic for recommendations prior to travel. It is a good idea for an INR to be checked as close to the time of departure as possible, especially if the trip will include a long car, train, or plane ride.

Before departing, individuals should know where they would seek emergency care at their destination. Their physician or anticoagulation clinic may have some suggestions.

For those individuals who are on a stable dose of warfarin and having their INR checked monthly, a trip out of town for up to a month does not present any problems. Individuals who are not on a stable dose of warfarin or who will be out of town for more than a month should make arrangements to have their INR checked while they are gone. In the United States, most communities have an urgent care facility. A provider there may be willing to order an INR test and communicate the results back to the patient's physician or anticoagulation clinic. In some foreign countries, medical laboratories may perform tests without a physician's order and fax or email the results to the patient's physician or anticoagulation clinic, which can then make recommendations regarding warfarin dosing.

Individuals who are not on a stable dose of warfarin or who will be out of town for more than a month should make arrangements to have their INR checked while they are gone.

Individuals who will be in extremely remote areas with limited resources may want to consider purchasing a coagulometer that uses test strips or cuvettes that do not require refrigeration. These patients can then seek guidance regarding warfarin dosing from their physician or anticoagulation clinic when communication allows. (See Question 36.)

PART TWELVE

Activity, Sports, and Recreation

What limitations do I have?

May I dive?

May I hike or climb?

More . . .

77. What limitations do I have?

One comforting thing about both DVT and PE is that they usually resolve successfully, allowing people to return to their previous activities. Two important issues should be considered with regard to sports and recreation, however. The first issue is the amount of clot present and the severity of leg pain or shortness of breath. The second issue is the potential for bleeding while you are being treated with an anticoagulant. Patients with very severe PE—bad enough to cause severe shortness of breath, fatigue, lightheadedness, fainting, or low oxygen levels—are unable to exercise initially, and their cases often take longer to resolve. For these patients, for patients with substantial leg pain and swelling, and for patients who have a very large clot in the leg or lung, bed rest for at least several days is recommended as treatment is delivered. Thus sports activity cannot be undertaken during this period.

Some physicians believe that *all* patients with DVT or PE should follow a bed rest regimen for at least several days after the initial event. Their concern is that if DVT is present, it may be more likely to break off (causing PE) if a patient stands and walks. Our extensive experience with outpatient treatment suggests that such a problem is actually very rare. Nevertheless, it is a good idea to remain on bed rest with the leg elevated for at least several days or longer while receiving treatment when large clots are present in the leg or when the leg is especially painful or swollen.

Once symptoms improve or when patients don't have significant initial symptoms from their DVT or PE, standing and walking are appropriate, although more vigorous exercise should be postponed for several weeks. People who enjoy participating in sports are well advised to wait several weeks to resume exercise, if this activity amounts to more than simply walking. Light weight training is also reasonable once initial symptoms subside. People with clots in their upper extremities (such as the arm or neck) would be wise to avoid vigorous arm exercise for several weeks and until their symptoms have significantly improved. It is important to realize that no research study results are available to guide any of these recommendations, so you should always follow your own physician's recommendations.

When you engage in any type of sports or recreation, be aware that anticoagulant medications such as warfarin (Coumadin®) increase your chances of bleeding and bruising. In general, people who are taking anticoagulants should avoid any activity involving a high risk of hard contact, especially head injury. They should not undertake physically demanding sports with the potential for contact or falling down, such as football or soccer.

There are no real dangers with sports or recreational activities such as bowling, dancing, or weightlifting, as long as the person taking an anticoagulant realizes that, for example, a heavy weight dropped on a foot or other body part could cause severe bruising or even a dangerous hematoma. Participation in other sports or recreation often depends on the level of exertion or aggression involved. Very demanding gymnastics could be very dangerous if the person suffers a fall, particularly one accompanied by a head injury. Fast-pitch softball or baseball could be extremely dangerous if a player on an anticoagulant was struck in the head. Kicking around a soccer ball, playing catch, or shooting baskets would be perfectly acceptable in a more relaxed setting. Riding a bicycle, skateboarding, or horseback riding might appear safe but would have to be done with caution. Martial arts training, including extremely cautious noncontact sparring, is reasonable; by contrast, boxing, unless it is also completely noncontact, must be avoided. A more aggressive level of activity involving any of these sports could, of course, be very dangerous.

Apart from the danger posed by an injury suffered while you are on an anticoagulant, your level of activity itself might be

DVT and PE usually resolve successfully, allowing people to return to their previous activities. Listen to your body while you are exercising, but recognize that immobility is an important risk factor for DVT and PE, so activity is important in preventing this problem.

limited by your symptoms related to a DVT or PE. Even a slow jog might be difficult in a previously healthy individual until his or her symptoms start to improve. A common saying that helps guide activity after DVT or PE is "Listen to your body." If shortness of breath or leg discomfort is particularly bothersome to you, slow down and rest. At the same time, immobility is an important risk factor for DVT and PE, so activity is important in preventing this problem! Even if you require oxygen, try to begin walking or exercise, if possible, once your initial symptoms have subsided.

Both DVT and PE can occasionally result in symptoms that either never go away or that come back again after they initially improve. When this happens, exercise can still be done as tolerated. Evaluation by a doctor is recommended in such a case, and additional testing may be needed.

78. May I dive?

If you want to scuba dive after experiencing DVT or PE, you should check with your physician to determine whether, depending on your overall health condition, this activity is safe. In general, there is no reason why you cannot eventually dive if your symptoms completely resolve and you do not require oxygen. However, you should not consider engaging in scuba diving until at least several months have passed. If your symptoms do not resolve, or especially if you have or develop pulmonary hypertension (high blood pressure in the lungs, which results in shortness of breath) after PE, you should not engage in diving.

Approximately one in five individuals has a **patent foramen ovale**—a hole in the heart separating its two upper chambers. Sometimes this condition is recognized during the evaluation for PE. If it is present, the risk of a blood clot going from the lung to the brain is increased, and diving could be dangerous.

79. May I hike or climb?

Several issues must be considered here. First, serious climbing at high altitudes requires that an individual's oxygen level be adequate. This level should always be checked, but particularly if the individual has had PE in the past. Second, individuals on anticoagulants are at very high risk for significant injury from a fall. Of course, such situations must be assessed on an individual basis. The danger of climbing, with regard to falling and bleeding, returns to baseline after anticoagulant therapy has been stopped.

Hiking is quite safe in general, but the individual's oxygen level should be checked to ensure that it is adequate after PE has occurred. Fitted elastic compression stockings are advised, particularly if the person is planning a long hike or vigorous walking. Such stockings may prevent leg swelling and more chronic leg problems.

Patent foreamen ovale

An opening in the partition that separates the upper two chambers of the heart, or atria. Such an opening can allow blood from the body to bypass the lungs and return to the body or brain. A blood clot in a person with a patent foreamen ovale could travel from the legs or other part of the body to the right side of the heart, through the patent foreamen ovale, bypass the lungs, travel through arteries, lodge in the brain and cause a stroke.

PART THIRTEEN

Complications

Can DVT cause permanent damage?

How can post-phlebitic or post-thrombotic syndrome be prevented?

What are the consequences of PE?

More . . .

80. Can DVT cause permanent damage?

Most patients recover from DVT without significant problems or complications, although occasionally longer-term problems may occur.

Most patients recover from DVT without significant problems or complications. Even patients who have very large clots with significant leg pain and swelling generally recover. Longer-term problems may occur, however.

The veins in the body have valves in them to keep blood flowing in the right direction. When a blood clot forms in the leg veins, it often forms around these valves. In some patients, the valves may become damaged so that the blood settles in the legs and doesn't move forward toward the heart as it should. Over months to years, this venous stasis (sluggish or nonexistent blood flow) may cause swelling in the legs and discoloration of the skin. Pain can develop as well. Of course, this post-phlebitic or post-thrombotic syndrome does not occur in everyone. (See Question 11.) It is variable in severity but can be quite disabling. Because of swelling and poor circulation, 10 to 20 percent of these patients develop ulcers in the skin, which sometimes require surgery.

Some patients develop these chronic problems without even having obvious DVT, presumably because the DVT was not associated with any symptoms when it occurred. That is, long-term problems may sometimes develop in patients who never even had their DVT diagnosed. Significant obesity may make these chronic leg problems even worse. Fitted elastic compression stockings may help to alleviate the symptoms from post-phlebitic syndrome.

Mike's story:

I am an executive with a large corporation, and I am responsible for major accounts worldwide. Currently, I am very active and coach competitive soccer, but I have to manage the consequences of DVT every day. The recurring pain in my calf and behind my knee limits my exercise and the activities that I can participate in.

I can't sit for long periods of time and have to be extremely careful on long flights.

I wish I had listened to my body when I could not control the swelling in my cast (pain means something). I wish I had known more about the risk factors for, and the signs of, DVT and PE when my problems began. I wish I had sought out the very best medical attention to immediately perform the lysis procedures on my leg as soon as the clots were detected. Unfortunately, wishing does not help. . . . DVTs and Coumadin® will always be a part of my life. I am lucky to have survived, and now I need to make major adjustments in my life going forward.

81. How can post-phlebitic or post-thrombotic syndrome be prevented?

You can reduce your risk of developing post-phlebitic or post-thrombotic syndrome by wearing fitted knee-high elastic compression stockings that exert a pressure of at least 30 to 40 mm Hg at the ankle with less pressure at the knee. While the duration for which they should be worn is unknown, their use for the first two years after a DVT is suggested.

82. What are the consequences of PE?

Pulmonary embolism does not result in complications in the vast majority of cases. Some people have just a few small emboli. Others, however, develop very large, massive clots that may block off the majority of the blood flow to the lung, causing dramatic symptoms, very low oxygen levels, and right heart failure. Because the right side of the heart—and particularly the right ventricle—has to pump blood into the lungs against a normally low pressure, the heart may not be able to keep up when there is a massive embolism in the lung and the right side of the heart may fail. (See Question 10.) In such a case, the person's blood pressure drops, and the heart may stop altogether. Thus the worst complication of PE is severe right heart failure and resulting death.

Pulmonary embolism does not result in complications in the vast majority of cases. If a patient survives the early hours after PE develops, he or she is likely to recover. The worst complication of PE is severe right heart failure and resulting death.

If a patient survives the early hours after PE develops, he or she is likely to recover. However, a recurrence can occur, which emphasizes the need for the patient to receive therapy as quickly as possible. When right heart failure does develop, as the clot resolves with treatment, the right heart returns to its previous state and functions normally (unless it was abnormal before the PE).

Sometimes pulmonary infarction can occur. This problem develops when a blood clot blocks a very small pulmonary artery that supplies a portion of the peripheral lung (outside edge of the lung). It causes pain and sometimes bleeding; the latter problem results in the person coughing up blood. While it may be painful, pulmonary infarction usually is associated with a smaller, less dangerous PE.

Sometimes, but particularly when pulmonary infarction has developed, a patient may develop fluid around the lung. These pleural effusions are usually small, but on rare occasions can be quite large, requiring drainage. This drainage can be done at the hospital bedside in nearly all cases, without surgery.

In some individuals, PE never completely resolves or actually gets worse over time. This outcome is unusual, affecting only 3 to 4 of every 100 individuals who develop an episode of PE.

83. Can PE cause permanent damage?

In some individuals, PE never completely resolves or actually gets worse over time. This outcome is unusual, affecting only 3 to 4 of every 100 individuals who develop an episode of PE.

In these individuals, the symptoms that occur during the initial episode of PE (such as shortness of breath or chest pain) usually resolve completely, and the person returns to his or her previous baseline health status. Over subsequent months (or usually years), however, the person may gradually develop shortness of breath as the damage from the initial PE progresses. The culprit here may be "silent," recurrent PE, or possibly growth of clots remaining in the lung.

Eventually, this problem may become severe enough that the person seeks medical attention. The diagnosis may be difficult to make but echocardiography (ultrasound pictures of the heart) may reveal high blood pressure in the lungs (pulmonary hypertension), which offers an important clue. Although either a VQ scan or CT scan can offer a more definitive diagnosis, often a catheterization test (a pulmonary arteriogram) gives the final answer. (See Question 14.)

This recurrent disease, which is known as chronic thromboembolic pulmonary hypertension (CTEPH), may cause very severe and disabling symptoms, or even death. The good news is that CTEPH is uncommon and can be cured in many cases with surgery. This specialized surgical procedure is performed at only a few centers in the United States and around the world, however. The University of California at San Diego has the most experience with this procedure. When the surgery is performed, the person's oxygen level generally improves significantly, the pulmonary hypertension resolves, and the right side of the heart is able to pump adequately again. In patients with CTEPH, an inferior vena caval filter is placed to prevent further clots from getting to the lungs (See Question 28) and warfarin therapy is continued.

84. How is swelling treated?

Swelling can result when the pressure inside of a vein or veins is higher than the pressure in the surrounding tissue, causing fluid to be forced out of the vein or veins and into the surrounding tissue. Pressure can increase in veins as a result of obstruction to blood flow from old clots or interference with forward blood flow from damaged valves (venous stasis). (See Question 80.) Any new leg swelling may be the result of new clot, so it should be evaluated by a physician.

Existing leg swelling is treated with fitted elastic compression stockings that exert 30 to 40 millimeters of mercury (mm Hg) pressure at the ankle. Fitted elastic compression stockings provide counter-pressure to veins and help return fluid that has leaked out of them back into the circulation. Elevating one's leg or legs can also help relieve swelling. If the person is overweight, weight loss can help. Diuretics ("water pills") are not effective and are not generally prescribed for the treatment of swelling due to venous stasis.

85. How is pain treated?

Besides swelling, people who have had a DVT can experience aching, heaviness, and pain in the affected leg. The most important treatment to reduce pain is to counteract the swelling with fitted elastic compression stockings. Elevating one's leg or legs can help. If the person is overweight, weight loss can help.

86. How are leg ulcers treated?

Why some people develop leg ulcers (that is, open sores) is not completely understood, but venous stasis (obstruction to blood flow from old clots or interference with forward blood flow from damaged valves) is almost always present. The signs of venous stasis include mild to severe swelling, aching, heaviness, pain, dilated superficial veins (varicose veins), a rusty discoloration of the skin caused by iron deposits from old blood, and sometimes ulcers.

Ulcers are treated with dressings that promote healing of the sore, fitted elastic compression stockings that improve circulation to the area, and, if necessary, surgery to remove dead tissue surrounding the ulcer. Ulcers can take weeks or months to heal. Elevating one's leg or legs can help. If the person is overweight, weight loss can help.

Recurrent blood clots are treated with anticoagulation and usually require lifelong therapy.

87. How are recurrent blood clots treated?

Recurrent blood clots are treated with anticoagulation (See Questions 16 and 23) and usually require lifelong therapy. Recurrent blood clots that occur while an individual is taking warfarin require investigation on the part of the physician or anticoagulation clinic to make sure that the warfarin dose is sufficient for the patient. Recurrent blood clots that occur despite a sufficient dose of warfarin require an alternative strategy. In such cases, LMWH or fondaparinux may be prescribed instead of warfarin. Individuals who have recurrent PE may require a vena caval filter. (See Question 28.)

PART FOURTEEN

Prevention of Recurrent Clots

What is the chance that I will
have another DVT or PE?

Should I avoid any specific foods or medications?

If I am not on anticoagulants, should
I take any special precautions?

More . . .

88. What is the chance that I will have another DVT or PE?

Your chance of having another DVT or PE depends on the circumstances surrounding your first DVT or PE. If your blood clot occurred as a result of surgery or trauma, and the risk factor was considered temporary, then your risk of having another DVT or PE may be very low. If your blood clot occurred spontaneously, without any risk factors being present, your risk of another clot is 30 percent over the next ten years. Obviously, your risk of having another DVT or PE will be higher if you have thrombophilia or cancer.

Sometimes, an ultrasound examination can provide information that can help the physician or anticoagulation clinic predict whether another blood clot will occur. Normal veins are less likely to develop recurrent clots than veins that contain residual clots.

89. Should I avoid any specific foods or medications?

Many people wonder whether vitamin K can cause blood clots, given that vitamin K is essential to the liver's production of the active forms of clotting factors II, VII, IX, and X. Vitamin K does not cause blood clots. In fact, no foods cause blood clots.

Conversely, several medications increase a person's risk of developing blood clots. Estrogen, and medications that have a similar chemical structure to estrogen, can increase the risk of blood clots. Estrogen is an ingredient in birth control pills, patches, and rings. It is also prescribed for the treatment of postmenopausal symptoms, including hot flushes and vaginal dryness. Medications that have a similar chemical structure to estrogen and increase the risk of blood clots include clomiphene citrate (Clomid®), which is used to treat female infertility, and tamoxifen, which is used to treat and prevent breast cancer. The hormones used to induce ovulation in women undergoing treatment for infertility can also increase the risk of blood clots.

While progestin, in the doses used in contraceptive pills (Micronor®, Nor-Q.D.®, Ovrette®), injections (Depo-Provera®), and the intrauterine device (Mirena®), has not been shown to increase the risk of DVT or PE, the higher doses used to treat abnormal vaginal bleeding have been shown to increase the risk of thrombosis five- to sixfold. Some newer cancer treatments that use thalidomide or thalidomide-like medications also increase patients' risk of blood clots.

90. If I am not on anticoagulants, should I take any special precautions?

Individuals who have experienced a DVT or PE in the past but are no longer on warfarin therapy should take the following precautions:

- Seek medical attention *immediately* if you develop pain or swelling in an arm or leg, shortness of breath, or chest pain.
- Always tell every doctor you see that you have a history of a blood clot.
- Walk for five minutes for every two hours you travel by car.
- If you plan an airplane flight lasting more than six hours, contact your doctor or your anticoagulation clinic for clot prevention recommendations.
- If you have elective surgery scheduled, contact your doctor or your anticoagulation clinic for clot prevention recommendations.
- For women: Do not take estrogen-containing medications, including estrogen-containing birth control pills, patches, or rings, or estrogen-containing pills or patches at menopause.

91. Does aspirin prevent blood clots?

Aspirin prevents platelets from becoming activated. (See Question 3.) This process is irreversible, so aspirin's effects can last for about a week, which is the lifespan of the affected platelets. By preventing platelets from becoming activated, aspirin keeps platelets from sticking to injured blood vessels.

Aspirin and other antiplatelet drugs, such as Plavix®, are very effective in preventing blood clots in the arteries—in other words, heart attacks and strokes—in people who have atherosclerosis (hardening of the arteries). Some studies show that these drugs also provide some protection against DVT and PE in people who are hospitalized; other studies have failed to confirm this effect, however. When aspirin was compared to other anticoagulants used to prevent DVT and PE in patients undergoing knee replacement or hip fracture surgery, the rate of blood clots in the aspirin group was double that in the group taking other anticoagulants. Aspirin may also increase a person's risk of bleeding, especially if it is used in conjunction with other anticoagulants. Aspirin does not provide sufficient protection against DVT and PE to allow it to be used as the only method to prevent DVT and PE.

PART FIFTEEN

Family and Genetic Issues

If I have had a blood clot, do I need to
be tested for thrombophilia?

If I learn that I have an inherited thrombophilia,
what should I tell my family members?

If I have a family member who has had a
blood clot or thrombophilia, but I have never
had a blood clot, what are my risks?

More . . .

92. If I have had a blood clot, do I need to be tested for thrombophilia?

There is controversy about exactly who should be tested for thrombophilia, so the answer to this question depends on the specific situation. Most experts agree that the following persons with thrombosis should be tested for thrombophilia:

- Younger individuals with a blood clot (age younger than 50 years)
- Individuals with a spontaneous blood clot
- Individuals with extensive blood clots or clots in an unusual location (for example, the veins of the brain or liver)
- Individuals with a blood clot who have family members who have had a DVT or PE
- Women who have had recurrent miscarriages or certain other pregnancy complications, such as babies with poor growth (fetal growth restriction), premature separation of the placenta from the uterus (placental abruption), preeclampsia (high blood pressure of pregnancy), or stillbirth

These individuals may undergo the tests listed in Table 1.

Table 1   Tests for Thrombophilia

Activated protein C resistance*	Prothrombin gene mutation
Antithrombin	Protein C
Protein S (activity and antigen levels)	Antiphospholipid antibody testing†
Homocysteine level	Factor VIII

* If activated protein C resistance is present, would also check for factor V Leiden.
† This generally includes testing for lupus anticoagulant and anticardiolipin antibodies.

93. If I learn that I have an inherited thrombophilia, what should I tell my family members?

Family members should be informed about both the thrombophilia in general and the specific condition (such as factor V Leiden or protein S deficiency). Family members who inherit the same genes may be at an increased risk of developing a DVT or PE. First-degree relatives (siblings, children, and parents) are at greater risk compared to extended family members (cousins, aunts, and uncles). Nevertheless, extended family members may benefit from this information as well. Family members should inform their healthcare providers of their potential for the inherited condition, and together they can decide whether testing is indicated.

It would be reasonable for family members who have had a blood clot in the past to be tested because the information might affect their treatment. For family members who have never developed a blood clot, testing should be done only after a discussion of what the information would mean for them.

94. If I have a family member who has had a blood clot or thrombophilia, but I have never had a blood clot, what are my risks?

Your risk may depend on whether you have inherited a tendency to form blood clots. As discussed earlier, clots can occur either sporadically or in response to certain risk factors (for example, trauma, pregnancy, and immobility). Another risk factor is related to your genes, including whether these genes, if inherited, might increase your susceptibility to developing a blood clot. Mutations within genes can be transmitted from generation to generation.

Thrombophilia is a predisposition to the development of blood clots that can result from mutations within genes. It can be either inherited or acquired during a person's lifetime.

If you discover that you have an inherited thrombophilia, you should inform family members about both the thrombophilia in general and your specific condition, because family members who inherit the same genes may be at an increased risk of developing a DVT or PE.

Inherited forms of thrombophilia are transmitted through genes and include factor V Leiden, prothrombin gene mutation, protein S deficiency, protein C deficiency, antithrombin deficiency, and some cases of elevated levels of homocysteine or factor VIII. There may be other inherited forms of thrombophilia that have not yet been discovered.

Inherited thrombophilia can increase a person's lifetime risk of a DVT or PE from 2 to 100 times. If an individual inherits one copy of a gene mutation, his or her risk of developing a blood clot is higher than normal. If an individual inherits two copies of a gene mutation (either the same mutation for an inherited thrombophilia or two different thrombophilias), his or her risk is much higher than normal.

95. If I have a family member who has had a blood clot or thrombophilia, but I have never had a blood clot, should I be tested for thrombophilia?

If the family member with a blood clot does not have an inherited thrombophilia, then it is less likely that the risk of a blood clot would be increased in other members of the family. In such a case, testing for thrombophilia would not be indicated. If it is not known whether the family member has an inherited (versus acquired) thrombophilia, then the healthcare provider would essentially have to perform a broad panel of tests to evaluate any unaffected family members. Without knowing which specific thrombophilia may or may not be present in the family member who had the blood clot, the results of a broad panel of tests may not be useful to other family members. Testing for thrombophilia, therefore, is not generally recommended in this situation.

If one of your first-degree relatives (sibling, child, or parent) has been diagnosed with an inherited thrombophilia, then you might want to discuss with your healthcare provider the option of being tested. This discussion should include which

INHERITANCE OF FACTOR V LEIDEN

When someone asks, "What are the chances of my child having this blood clotting disorder?" the answer depends on the type of thrombophilia that the patient has. The following examples describe specific situations related to the most common inherited thrombophilia, factor V Leiden:

If a person is homozygous for factor V Leiden (in other words, if the person has two copies of the factor V Leiden gene), each of his or her children will be heterozygous for factor V Leiden at the very least (in other words, each child will have one copy of the factor V Leiden gene). A child could be homozygous for factor V Leiden *only* if the other parent also has the factor V Leiden gene.

If a person is heterozygous for factor V Leiden, then each of his or her children has a 50-50 chance of being heterozygous for factor V Leiden. Depending on the other parent's genetic makeup, a child could have no factor V Leiden, could be heterozygous for factor V Leiden, or could even be homozygous for factor V Leiden.

If a person does not have factor V Leiden, then his or her children will inherit only normal factor V genes from that parent. Factor V Leiden does not "skip" generations.

specific tests would be done, what the likelihood of a positive test result would be, what a positive result would mean for you and your family, and, if a test is positive, what changes in lifestyle or treatments you should consider.

For people who test positive, additional issues would likely need to be discussed after the results are obtained. In addition, consultation with a genetic counselor might be appropriate.

A genetic counselor can assess risks based on family history, provide education about the condition in question, and describe the risks, benefits, and limitations of testing.

Whether an individual decides to pursue testing is a personal choice. Some people decide to undergo testing because the results may help them make certain lifestyle changes or seek treatment. For example, a woman who tests positive for an inherited thrombophilia might choose to avoid oral contraceptives or estrogen therapy. Some people who test positive might choose to take an aspirin a day, although studies have not proved that this measure will prevent a venous blood clot (See Question 91). For some individuals, simply knowing that they have a negative test result might provide peace of mind.

Other people may choose to decline testing because the information may not be useful to them. As with any inherited or genetic condition, there may be some concern about potential health or life insurance discrimination. The risk of being denied or having to pay higher premiums for coverage is not well regulated.

If you are interested in being tested, you should speak to your primary care provider or seek out a genetic counselor who is knowledgeable about bleeding and clotting disorders.

PART SIXTEEN

Miscellaneous Topics

Do I need to wear a medical identification bracelet or necklace?

What does insurance usually pay for?

Who treats DVT and PE?

More . . .

96. Do I need to wear a medical identification bracelet or necklace?

Wearing a medical identification bracelet or necklace is an excellent idea if you are taking warfarin. Such an identifier can alert emergency medical personnel that you are on warfarin and should be worn continuously. Emergency medical personnel do pay attention to such jewelry.

"Warfarin" can be engraved on the surface of this bracelet or necklace. In addition, any other information that would be important in an emergency—such as other medications, medical conditions, and allergies—should be engraved there as well. Emergency contacts (next of kin, physician) and other information can be included as space permits. Additional information can be carried on a card in a wallet or purse.

As a precaution, your physician or other healthcare provider should approve what will be engraved the medical identification tag. Order forms can be obtained from a physician's office or anticoagulation clinic or be downloaded from the Internet.

97. What does insurance usually pay for?

Insurance typically pays for physician fees, the costs of diagnostic procedures, and hospitalizations. While visits with physicians are covered, a copayment may be required for each visit. With frequent monitoring of the INR, the cost of these copayments can add up.

Although most insurance plans pay for medications, the copayment may be higher for brand-name Coumadin® than for generic warfarin. While there should be little, if any, difference between generic warfarin and Coumadin®, some physicians and anticoagulation clinics prefer that their patients take the brand-name product. The concern is that any variation between different formulations of warfarin could affect an individual's INR. Even for those patients who take generic warfarin all the time, there is no assurance that warfarin from the same manufacturer will be used each time a prescription is filled. Taking brand-name Coumadin®, instead of generic warfarin, may provide more consistency.

During the initial treatment of DVT or PE, insurance plans pay for low-molecular-weight heparin (LMWH) or fondaparinux until warfarin takes effect. Insurance plans also pay for LMWH during pregnancy. Sometimes they may be reluctant to pay for long-term therapy with LMWH or fondaparinux for other indications. In such a case, the physician or anticoagulation clinic may have to contact a medical director at the insurance plan and explain why a patient requires an anticoagulant other than warfarin. Even if the insurance plan approves another anticoagulant, the copayment for LMWH or fondaparinux may be quite expensive.

Medicare, Medicaid, and most insurance plans will not pay for coagulometers for patients, unless the insured person has a mechanical heart valve.

98. Who treats DVT and PE?

Depending on the severity of their initial condition, patients with DVT or PE may be treated by several different kinds of providers. Patients who present to their primary care doctor or to an emergency department with an uncomplicated DVT may be completely treated on an outpatient basis, starting with LMWH or fondaparinux therapy and then converting to warfarin. Patients with a more extensive clot, with a clot in an unusual location (for example, in the veins in the abdomen or in the head), or with other conditions that might predispose them to bleeding, however, are more likely to be admitted to the hospital for their initial treatment. Some studies indicate that patients with an uncomplicated PE may also be treated as outpatients, but many physicians are more likely to admit these patients to the hospital for their initial treatment.

Patients who are being considered for thrombolytic drugs because of a life-threatening PE will usually be evaluated by a pulmonary specialist for initial treatment (See Question 29). If the patient is being considered for a vena caval filter (See Question 28) or use of a new device that breaks up clots while simultaneously injecting a thrombolytic drug into the clot (See Question 29), then an interventional radiologist—a radiologist with special training in these procedures—will also be involved.

After initial treatment, when the patient's condition is stable and he or she is taking only warfarin, the individual may be cared for by his or her primary physician, or by an anticoagulation clinic, which may be staffed by a pharmacist or a nurse. If the person is found to have a thrombophilia, he or she might be referred to a hematologist. After six months of anticoagulation therapy, the person might also be referred to a specialist to review all of the laboratory tests and the course of treatment to determine whether a longer course of treatment is necessary.

Some patients with DVT and PE may develop chronic complications that require treatment by a specialist. For example, a person who develops post-phlebitic syndrome may need to see a dermatologist or other provider who specializes in treatment of chronic leg swelling (See Question 84). If a person with a massive PE develops pulmonary hypertension (See Question 83), he or she may need to see a pulmonary specialist.

99. Where can I find an expert in the field?

Depending on your individual situation, an "expert" in the field can be any of several different people:

• If an individual needs someone to monitor warfarin therapy, an "expert" would be a provider in a dedicated anticoagulation clinic. You can find a list of anticoagulation clinics designated by region at the Anticoagulation Forum Web site (www.acforum.org).

- Most pediatricians who take care of children with clots are trained as pediatric hematologists and will be located in a university or other major medical center. They would work with a local pediatrician to manage the child's warfarin therapy.

- If the patient is a woman who is pregnant or thinking about becoming pregnant, she should see an obstetrician who specializes in high-risk pregnancies. Obstetricians with experience in the care of women with thrombophilia or a history of thrombosis are more likely to be affiliated with hemostasis and thrombosis referral centers.

- If the individual has an inherited thrombophilia or is interested in being tested for an inherited thrombophilia, he or she should see a provider who specializes in thrombophilia. This provider could be a hematologist, a cardiologist, a pulmonary specialist, or a general internist, depending on the particular community. A genetics counselor could also provide useful insights into inherited thrombophilia.

- If a patient on chronic anticoagulation needs a surgical procedure, a team approach is important: the surgeon must work with the providers who will manage the anticoagulation therapy. In some cases, a patient might need low-molecular-weight heparin while warfarin is stopped, or possibly placement of an inferior vena caval filter, which needs to be coordinated with the surgeon.

100. Where can I go for additional information?

About Lovenox® (Enoxaparin)

This Web site has information about blood clots, the dangers of DVT, and methods of anticoagulation: www.lovenox.com/consumer/aboutLovenox/main.aspx.

American College of Chest Physicians

The American College of Chest Physicians (ACCP) is a medical specialty society of physicians, surgeons, other health professionals, and individuals with Ph.D. degrees who specialize in diseases of the chest. Since 1986, it has published guidelines about antithrombotic and thrombolytic therapy. These guidelines are now published approximately every three years. The current guidelines, "The Seventh ACCP Conference on Antithrombotic and Thrombolytic Therapy: Evidence-Based Guidelines," were published in September 2004 in a supplement to the medical journal *Chest*. These guidelines, while directed at physicians and other healthcare providers, provide a thorough and up-to-date summary of the optimal treatment and prevention of DVT and PE. The next ACCP statement will be published in 2007.

APS Foundation of America

The APS Foundation of America is an organization that was founded to provide support and education to people with antiphospholipid antibody syndrome (a rare thrombotic disorder associated with recurrent thromboembolism), as well as their friends and family members. Its Web site is located at www.apsfa.org

Cardiology Patient Page

The medical journal *Circulation* occasionally publishes articles specifically for patients. These articles, which are written by world-renowned experts, have been compiled on the Cardiology Patient Page (http://circ.ahajournals.org/collected/patient.shtml). Titles include "Heparin-Induced Thrombocytopenia," "Antiphospholipid Antibodies," "Homocysteine and MTHFR Mutations: Relation to Thrombosis and Coronary Artery Disease," "Prevention of Deep Vein Thrombosis and Pulmonary Embolism," "Prothrombin 20210 Mutation (Factor II Mutation)," "Factor V Leiden," "Pulmonary Hypertension," "Treatment of Blood Clots," "Diseases of the Veins," and "Pulmonary Embolism and Deep Vein Thrombosis."

Coalition to Prevent Deep Vein Thrombosis

The Coalition to Prevent Deep Vein Thrombosis is sponsored by Sanofi-Aventis Corporation. The mission of this organization is to reduce the immediate- and long-term dangers of DVT and PE. The coalition serves to educate the public, healthcare professionals, and policy makers about risk factors, symptoms, and signs associated with DVT, as well as to identify measures to prevent morbidity and mortality from DVT and PE. More information is available on its Web site (www.preventdvt.org/).

Coumadin.com

The Coumadin® Web site has information for patients about warfarin. Its address is www.coumadin.com.

DVT.NET

DVT.NET is a Web site sponsored by Sanofi-Aventis Corporation, which manufactures Lovenox®, a low-molecular-weight heparin. The Web site (www.dvt.net/) provides information about DVT, risk factors, symptoms, and protective measures that can be taken to reduce the risk of blood clots.

Fragmin® (Dalteparin) Patient Home Page

The Web site for the low-molecular-weight heparin, dalteparin (Fragmin®), has information on blood clots, risk factors, complications of blood clots, prevention of blood clots, and the drug dalteparin. Its address is www.fragmin.com/patient/patient_home.asp.

FVL Thrombophilia Support Page

This Web site is hosted by an individual who has factor V Leiden. It contains information for patients and patient stories. The Web address is www.fvleiden.org/.

Innohep® (Tinzaparin) USA Web Site

The Innohep® USA Web site has information about DVT, the dual diagnosis of DVT and cancer, management of

DVT, tinzaparin, and important safety information. Its address is www.innohepusa.com/corporateweb/innohepus/home.nsf/Content/Home-Consumer.

National Alliance for Thrombosis and Thrombophilia

An excellent source for information that is both up-to-date and accurate is the National Alliance for Thrombosis and Thrombophilia (NATT). NATT is a nationwide, community-based, volunteer health organization that was formed in August 2003. It is committed to preventing and treating the array of major health problems caused by blood clots. Its goal is to ensure that people suffering from thrombosis and thrombophilia get early diagnosis, optimal treatment, and quality support. NATT members are committed to fostering research, education, support, and advocacy on behalf of those at risk of, or affected by, blood clots.

A primary goal of NATT is to provide education and information to individuals and families affected by blood clots and blood clotting disorders. The organization is currently developing its own materials to address these topics. In the meantime, members of the Education Committee have identified and reviewed published materials in subject areas relevant to individuals and families affected by blood clots and clotting disorders. A list of these published materials can be found on the NATT Web site at www.nattinfo.org/learn.htm. The materials were required to meet the following criteria before they could be added to this list:

- Be informative
- Be written in language that is understandable
- Be accurate
- Be up-to-date
- Be hosted by a reputable organization (such as a university health center or government health organization)
- Be peer-reviewed (meaning that the material is reviewed by other healthcare providers and/or patients before its publication)

- Be accessible—on the Internet and often as a PDF or printable version

We encourage you to visit the NATT Web site and consider joining the organization.

United States Centers for Disease Control and Prevention

The Division of Hereditary Blood Disorders of the U.S. Centers for Disease Control and Prevention (CDC) is helping to establish a network of hemostasis and thrombosis centers to promote the management, treatment, and prevention of complications experienced by persons with clotting disorders and is conducting laboratory work to identify genetic risk factors that predispose persons to thrombophilia. Identifying these factors could help prevent complications that result from clotting. More information for individuals with clotting disorders is available on the CDC's Web site at www.cdc. gov/ncbddd/hbd/clotting.htm.

United States Department of Agriculture

Information about the vitamin K content of various foods is available on the U.S. Department of Agriculture (USDA) Web site. Two documents are available there: "USDA National Nutrient Database for Standard Reference, Release 18—Vitamin K (Phylloquinone) (µg) Content of Selected Foods per Common Measure, Sorted by Nutrient Content" and "USDA National Nutrient Database for Standard Reference, Release 18—Vitamin K (Phylloquinone) (µg) Content of Selected Foods per Common Measure, Sorted Alphabetically." These documents can be found at www.ars.usda. gov/Services/docs.htm?docid=9673.

United States Food and Drug Administration

The U.S. Food and Drug Administration (FDA) provides consumer information on anticoagulants on its Web site (www.fda.gov/cder).

Glossary

A

Acquired: A condition that is not genetic (inherited) or congenital (present at birth); usually caused by environmental factors and/or other physical conditions.

Activated partial thromboplastin time (aPTT): A blood test that measures the length of time (in seconds) that it takes for clotting to occur when certain substances are added to the liquid portion of blood in a test tube. The aPTT is used not only to detect clotting factor deficiencies, but also used to monitor heparin's effectiveness.

Anemia: A low red blood cell count. Anemia may be due to many causes, including low iron stores (called "iron-deficiency anemia") or antibody-mediated destruction of red blood cells (referred to as "autoimmune hemolytic anemia").

Antibody: A protein produced by the immune system in the body that travels in the blood and helps the body fight infection.

Anticoagulant: A type of medication that causes the blood to take a longer time to form a blood clot. Anticoagulants are used to prevent formation of blood clots and to treat blood clots once they develop. These drugs may be given by injection, either into a vein or under the skin (e.g., heparin, low-molecular-weight heparin), or by mouth (warfarin).

Anticoagulation: A general term for a treatment that interferes with the ability of the blood to form a normal blood clot. Anticoagulant medicines include heparin and warfarin, and are sometimes referred to as "blood thinners."

Antiphospholipid antibody: A type of autoantibody (an antibody directed against one's own tissues) associated with an increased risk for forming blood clots (deep vein thrombosis, pulmonary embolism, stroke, and heart attack) or recurrent miscarriages. These autoantibodies generally do not bind directly to phospholipids, but instead bind to certain proteins that in turn bind to phospholipids.

Antiphospholipid antibody syndrome (APS): A rare autoimmune disorder characterized by recurrent blood clots and/or miscarriages. By definition, people with APS have elevated antiphospholipid antibody levels in their blood. APS may occur in individuals with lupus or related autoimmune diseases, or as a primary syndrome in otherwise healthy individuals (referred to as "primary APS").

Arterial blood gas (ABG): A technique used primarily to measure the oxygen level of blood with precision. It is obtained directly from an artery with a needle or a thin tube (catheter).

Artery: A vessel through which the blood passes away from the heart and to the various parts of the body.

Atrial fibrillation: An abnormal rhythm or heartbeat pattern involving the atria or the upper chambers of the heart (as opposed to the ventricles or lower chambers of the heart). The abnormal rhythm can interrupt the normal flow of blood through the heart, allowing clots to form that can then travel through arteries, lodge in the brain, and cause strokes.

Autoantibody: An antibody directed against one's own tissues.

B

Blood: A bodily fluid that circulates in the arteries and veins. Blood consists of plasma (the liquid portion that contains proteins and other molecules) and cells. Blood cells include white blood cells, which fight infection; red blood cells, which carry oxygen to the tissues and carbon dioxide back to the lungs; and platelets, which are like little corks that plug up holes to stop bleeding.

Budd-Chiari syndrome: Thrombosis of the hepatic veins (veins coming from the liver), usually presenting with abdominal pain, enlargement of the liver, and ascites (fluid in the abdomen).

C

Chronic thromboembolic pulmonary hypertension (CTEPH): High blood pressure in the lungs that occurs in a small percentage of patients who have had pulmonary embolism. The most common symptom is shortness of breath. This problem usually progresses but may be cured with surgery.

Clot: A thrombus.

Coagulation: The process of blood clotting.

Coagulometer: A device used to measure the INR for warfarin monitoring. Devices that can be used at home are available.

Coumadin®: Brand name for warfarin.

D

D-dimer: A breakdown product of fibrin, which is present in a blood clot. D-dimers are not generally present in the blood unless a clot has begun to form, although the presence of D-dimers does not guarantee that a clot is present. If D-dimers are absent, it is very unlikely that a blood clot has begun to form.

Deep vein thrombosis (DVT): A condition in which a blood clot forms in the deep veins of the legs, pelvis, or arms. The treatment for DVT includes anticoagulant therapy.

E

Endothelium: The lining of a blood vessel. Damage to the endothelium, such as from trauma (or a previous blood clot), makes a patient more susceptible to a blood clot.

Estrogen: A female hormone that occurs naturally, helps sustain pregnancy, and can be synthesized. It is a key ingredient in birth control pills, patches, and rings, and in postmenopausal hormone therapy.

F

Factor V Leiden: Factor V is an important blood clotting protein. Factor V Leiden occurs when a specific mutation in the factor V gene results in a protein that is more resistant to being turned off, leading to an increased risk for forming blood clots. Factor V Leiden is the most common inherited hypercoagulable state or thrombophilia.

Fibrin: A solid substance formed from fibrinogen, a specialized protein or clotting factor that is found in blood. Fibrin makes a clot more stable (harder to break up). It forms the mesh or net that holds blood platelets firmly in place.

Fibrinogen: A specialized protein or clotting factor that is found in blood. When a blood vessel is injured, another clotting factor, thrombin, is activated and converts fibrinogen to fibrin, which is the mesh or net that holds platelets firmly in place.

Fitted elastic compression stockings: Elastic stockings, which ideally exert a pressure of at least 30 to 40 mm Hg at the ankle with less pressure at the knee. Fitted elastic compression stockings provide counter-pressure to veins and help return fluid that has leaked out of them back into the circulation.

Fresh frozen plasma: The quickest way to reverse warfarin is to replace clotting factors. This is done with fresh frozen plasma; plasma is the liquid portion of blood that contains the clotting factors.

G

Gene: The blueprints for making individual proteins, located in the DNA. The human genome codes for an estimated 20,000 to 25,000 individual genes.

H

Hematologist: A physician who specializes in the study of blood disorders, such as bleeding and clotting problems, anemia, thrombocytopenia (a low number of platelets), and white blood cell disorders.

Hemoglobin: The protein molecule in red blood cells that carries oxygen from the lungs to the body's tissues and returns carbon dioxide from the tissues to the lungs. The iron contained in hemoglobin is responsible for the red color of blood.

Heparin: An anticoagulant medicine ("blood thinner") that is routinely prescribed for the treatment of clotting disorders, including treatment of clots in the coronary arteries (causing heart attack), clots in the blood vessels of the brain (leading to stroke), clots that occur in leg veins (deep vein thrombosis), and clots that obstruct blood flow to the lungs (pulmonary emboli).

Hypercoagulable: Refers to an increased tendency to form blood clots, due to either an inherited state (for example, factor V Leiden) or an acquired disorder (for example, cancer).

Hypercoagulable state: An inherited or acquired risk for developing blood clots. Common inherited causes of blood clots include factor V Leiden and the prothrombin gene mutation G20210A. Common acquired causes of blood clots include pregnancy, certain medications (for example, birth control pills), and cancer.

Hypertension: High blood pressure.

I

International normalized ratio (INR): A measurement of the blood's ability to clot based on the prothrombin time. In a normal individual, the INR should be 1. In a patient taking warfarin therapy, the blood takes longer to form a clot in a test tube, and the INR will be higher. The desired INR for many individuals taking warfarin is in the range of 2 to 3, but some individuals with antiphospholipid syndrome are maintained at a higher INR.

L

Low-molecular-weight heparin (LMWH): Chemically cut or cleaved heparin. LMWH lasts longer, must be monitored differently, and generally has fewer side effects than standard heparin.

Lupus: An autoimmune disorder characterized by multiple types of autoantibodies. Common clinical manifestations include arthritis, facial rashes, and fatigue. Many patients

with lupus will have antiphospholipid antibodies, referred to as secondary antiphospholipid syndrome.

Lupus anticoagulant: A type of antiphospholipid antibody that is detected through blood clotting tests, especially the activated partial thromboplastin time (aPTT). This autoantibody is associated with an increased risk for blood clots.

Lyse or **lysis:** To lyse a clot is to dissolve or destroy a clot. Lysis is the process whereby a clot is dissolved or destroyed. This process can occur naturally over time or can be accomplished by powerful, clot-busting drugs (thrombolytics).

M

Magnetic resonance imaging (MRI): A test that images clots in the body. While MRI does a better job of imaging the veins in the pelvis, abdomen, and chest than ultrasound does, ultrasound for the legs is usually adequate (and is cheaper). Neither test exposes a patient to radiation.

Mutation: A change in a gene from its natural state. Mutations may cause disease or result in a normal variant that causes no problems for the patient.

P

Patent foreamen ovale: An opening in the partition that separates the upper two chambers of the heart, or atria. Such an opening can allow blood from the body to bypass the lungs and return to the body or brain. A blood clot in a person with a patent forea-men ovale could travel from the legs or other part of the body to the right side of the heart, through the pat-ent foreamen ovale, bypass the lungs, travel through arteries, lodge in the brain and cause a stroke.

Phospholipid: A type of fat molecule found in many locations throughout the body, including in the membranes that surround all of our cells.

Plasma: The liquid part of the blood, which contains all the proteins neces-sary to form a blood clot, antibodies, and a variety of other components.

Plasminogen: A substance naturally produced by the body that helps to break down blood clots. The active form of plasminogen is called plasmin.

Platelet: The smallest cell in the blood. Platelets are important for normal blood clotting; they prevent blood from leaking out of an injured blood vessel.

Polycythemia: Too many red blood cells. If severe, polycythemia may predispose a patient to DVT.

Post-phlebitic (post-thrombotic) syndrome: Long-term, recurring leg symptoms that affect some patients as a result of permanent injury to veins and their valves from DVT.

Proteins: Essential molecules in the body that are made up of strings of amino acids. The genes in our DNA contain the necessary information to make all the proteins in our bodies. Examples of proteins include antibod-ies and blood clotting factors.

Prothrombin: A protein in the blood that is essential for the formation of a blood clot. The active form of pro-thrombin is called thrombin.

Prothrombin gene G20210A muta-tion: An abnormality of the gene for the clotting factor, prothrombin, lo-cated at position 20210, that results in the production of more prothrombin. In individuals with this prothrombin gene mutation, prothrombin levels are higher, contributing to increased formation of blood clots.

Prothrombin time (PT): A measure of how long it takes blood to clot in a test tube. This blood test is very sensi-tive to the effects of warfarin, vitamin K deficiency, or liver disease.

Pulmonary angiogram: The most definitive test to diagnose PE. Pulmo-nary angiogram is an "invasive" test, requiring injection of a dye through a catheter (IV line) into the body. Be-cause newer tests such as CT scans are now available, pulmonary angiography is rarely needed today.

Pulmonary artery: The main blood vessel carrying blood from the right side of the heart (right ventricle) into the lungs to pick up oxygen. This large blood vessel divides into smaller and smaller branches deeper into the lung. The pulmonary arteries are where pul-monary emboli migrate to and become lodged.

Pulmonary embolism (PE): A blood clot from a deep vein, usually in the legs, pelvis, or arms, that breaks loose and travels through the veins and then through the heart before becoming lodged in the blood vessels in the lung. Large pulmonary emboli can be life-threatening and may need to be treated with thrombolytic drugs ("clot-busters").

Pulmonary infarction: Pulmonary embolism that occurs in a small, dead-end pulmonary artery, resulting in the death of a small area of lung. It often causes pain in the chest or back.

Pulse oximetry: A noninvasive (no blood needed!) method of monitoring the percentage of hemoglobin that is saturated with oxygen. A low saturation may be caused by a number of lung or heart diseases, including pulmonary embolism.

R

Red blood cell: A cell in the blood that carries oxygen to the tissues. Red blood cells are an important component of blood clots.

S

Spontaneous DVT: A clot that forms when there are no obvious risk factors. Twenty to 40 percent of people who develop a spontaneous DVT have an inherited or acquired predisposition to thrombosis or thrombophilia.

Superficial thrombophlebitis: A blood clot or clots that form in the veins nearer to the surface.

T

Thrombin: The clotting factor that converts fibrinogen to fibrin.

Thrombocytopenia: A low platelet count.

Thrombocytosis (thrombocythemia): Too many blood platelets. It may predispose a patient to thrombosis.

Thrombophilia: A predisposition to the development of blood clots. It is sometimes referred to as "hypercoagulability." Thrombophilia can be either inherited or acquired during a person's lifetime.

Thrombosis: The pathologic (abnormal) process whereby liquid blood forms a clot within a blood vessel or the heart.

Thrombus: A blood clot.

Tissue factor: A substance that is released from the blood vessel lining and initiates the clotting reaction.

U

Ulcer: A chronic (long-standing) open sore.

Ultrasound: A test used to identify a number of medical conditions. When DVT is suspected, the inability to compress the leg veins with the ultrasound device indicates the presence of DVT. Abnormal blood flow can also be demonstrated when DVT is present.

V

Varicose veins: Enlarged, prominent veins that result from damaged valves.

Vein: A vessel through which blood passes from various organs back to the heart.

Vena cava: A large vein that carries blood to the heart, and then on to the lungs to pick up oxygen. The "superior" branch of the vena cava carries blood from the upper part of the body; the "inferior" branch of the vena cava carries blood from the lower part of the body.

Vena caval filter: A device inserted to prevent PE in patients with DVT and/or PE when anticoagulants fail or cannot be used.

Vitamin K: A vitamin that is essential to the production of the active forms of clotting factors II, VII, IX, and X in the liver.

Virchow's triad: The three basic factors that increase a patient's risk for deep vein thrombosis: (1) stasis (reduced mobility or immobility), (2) injury to a blood vessel, and (3) hypercoagulability.

VQ lung scan: A test to evaluate both air flow (V = ventilation) and blood flow (Q = perfusion) in the lungs to determine whether a person has experienced a pulmonary embolism.

W

Warfarin: A medicine given by mouth that interferes with blood clotting and is generally used for the prevention or treatment of blood clots. It is often referred to as a "blood thinner."

INDEX

Index